Your MediRoots Gui
to Medical C

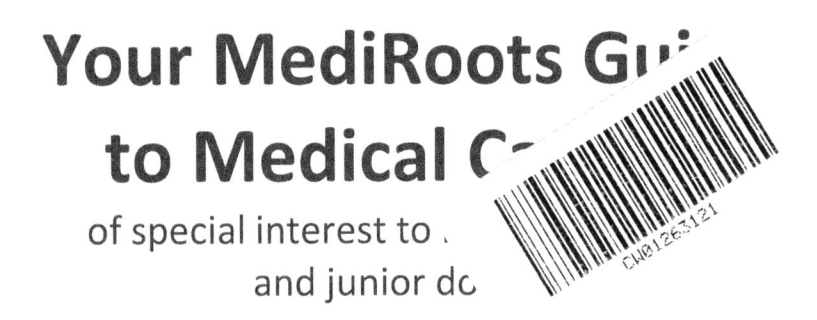

of special interest to
and junior do

Dr Yazdan Zargham

Dr Ruth Chambers

Eleanor Scott

Copyright

© Dr Yazdan Zargham and Dr Ruth Chambers have asserted their rights under the Copyright, Designs and Patents Act 1988 to be identified as the authors of this work. All rights reserved. No part of this publication may be reproduced, stored in a retrieval system or transmitted, in any form or by any means, electronic, mechanical, photocopying, recording or otherwise, without the prior permission of the copyright owner.

Cover and cartoons by John Byrne.

Date of publication - September 2021

Thanks

Thanks to Paula Stather for editing and designing the handbook content ready for publication; thanks to Chris Chambers for his 'back office' work too.

Disclaimer

All the guidance, ideas and suggestions included in the content of this medical careers handbook are intended to inform readers about how to optimize their experience and skills, and balance their needs and preferences in planning and pursuing their own medical career.
The content is not a substitute for national advice and guidance from professional or regulatory organizations that is constantly being updated. Whilst every effort has been made to include accurate and up to date information, updates in the delivery of medical specialties are constantly evolving – for example the accelerated digital transformation of health care during the COVID pandemic. So you need to use the content of this handbook to learn more about how you can think out your medical career options and weigh up the choices, and use the information and guidance for your own circumstances. Inclusion of named agencies, websites, companies, services or publications in this book does not constitute a recommendation or endorsement by the authors.

Contents

Authors   1

Preface   2

Abbreviations   4

Chapter 1   So many medical career paths - which/why/when/ how?   7

Chapter 2   The UK context for medical specialty training of junior doctors   19

Chapter 3   Get familiar with the range of medical specialty training pathways: 24
- anaesthetics   27
- clinical radiology   32
- general practice   37
- general surgery   41
- internal medicine   51
- obstetrics and gynaecology   56
- paediatrics   61
- palliative medicine   67
- psychiatry   73
- public health   80
- international medical graduates   86

Chapter 4   Prepare for your specialty interview   93

Chapter 5   Making a career choice   103

Chapter 6   Career planning   116

Chapter 7   Reflect on your progress as a qualified doctor and plan your career – yourself   125

Chapter 8   Get ready, set, go...............   148

About the authors

Dr Yazdan Zargham MBBS

Yazdan is a GP trainee in the Northwest of England, after completing his Foundation training at Royal Stoke and Queen's Burton Hospitals. Yazdan completed his medical training in Armenia, after which he came to practise in the UK. After struggling to decide on a chosen specialty career path as a junior Foundation doctor, Yazdan is very enthusiastic and passionate about helping medical students and other junior doctors to make informed decisions regarding their future careers. This is something Yazdan hopes to lead on and develop in future work and projects.

Professor Ruth Chambers OBE, FRCGP, DM

Ruth is an honorary professor at Staffordshire University and Keele University after an extensive academic medical career that has included research, education and at scale quality management in the NHS. Her career included a stint as Director of Postgraduate General Practice Education for the West Midlands. Until recently she was Clinical Chair of Stoke-on-Trent Clinical Commissioning Group and recently retired as a practising GP after 40+ years as a medic at the frontline. Ruth was a clinical lead for digital primary care transformation across Staffordshire. Ruth has written 76 books – mainly for doctors and health care teams, some for the public on health matters. She has presented at local events, national & international conferences; as well as carrying out research on doctors' work stress, contributing to national guidance such as rebutting prescription fraud, and extensive teaching of doctors and other health professionals at all stages of their careers.

Eleanor Scott RGN, BA (Hons), MSc

Eleanor is currently a PhD student at Keele University, focusing on Video Group Consultation in primary care general practice.
After completing a BA in Religious Studies at Lancaster University in 2016, Eleanor began an MSc in Adult Nursing at Keele University (2017-2019). Whilst working on Intensive Care as a Staff Nurse at Royal Stoke University Hospital, Eleanor is completing her PhD alongside her clinical practice. She has a great interest in the future of the workforce underpinning primary care, academia and service improvement, upon which this handbook is focused.

Preface

This handbook will provide medical students and doctors in their Foundation training years or at other stages of their specialty training programmes with careers information and advice, where pathway choices have to be made as their career evolves. We share information about ten medical specialty pathways, including what clinical areas each specialty covers, guidance on entry requirements and making a successful application.

Many doctors describe the paucity of careers support available to them as medical students, as doctors in training and for established doctors too – to enable them to make the right career choices that match their personality, interests, hopes and circumstances. Challenging doctors and medical students to review their own situation, formulate career aspirations and plan their career track is key to them enjoying and flourishing in their medical careers and sustaining their job satisfaction. Putting them back in touch with the values and beliefs that brought them into medicine and providing opportunities to diversify and develop, should help to retain doctors in practice long-term.

This handbook signposts the reader to short videoed conversations of many experienced doctors who are now practising in consultant or equivalent roles in a range of medical specialties and how they have made it along their career paths in such a variety of ways - see the **MediRoots** website (https://www.mediroots.co.uk).

These doctors describe their many diverse careers and achievements, discuss the nature of their work, the pros and cons, and share their insights about career choice and progression from their personal experiences. The content of each interview follows the lines along which the person being interviewed wanted to take the conversation. Doctors starring on the MediRoots site represent a breadth of age, gender and careers experience.

This resource will provide junior doctors and medical students with a wide range of 'stories' of success that they can apply to their own circumstances - giving them confidence that they can emulate one or more of the achievers interviewed in line with their own personal circumstances & potential– whatever their age or ethnicity, whatever education they have had or situation that they are in.
They'll get engaging tips on how to apply what the achievers have done from the advice and wisdom that they share in their interviews,
to optimise the viewer's likelihood of a successful career too.

You Can Do It Too!

The purpose of the **MediRoots** website (https://www.mediroots.co.uk) and this accompanying handbook is to provide medical students and junior doctors with guidance and support in informing their decisions regarding specialty career choices. Junior doctors are required to make their career decisions with limited experience and knowledge with regards to certain specialties, which can be a very daunting challenge for some.

So we hope that this handbook will help to:
- educate medical students and junior doctors and familiarise them with the range of medical specialties
- reduce specialty 'drop-out' when medical students and junior doctors make an *informed* choice regarding their career pathway and feel *confident* to diversify along the way
- increase the number of committed doctors in their chosen specialty
- extend medical students' and junior doctors' perspectives about portfolio careers, and the variety of career paths that are associated with particular medical specialties
- enhance awareness of how career planning tools can help doctors to review and align their medical career pathways to fit their strengths, needs and preferences.

Abbreviations

ACCS	Acute Care Common Stem
ATLS	Advanced Trauma Life Support
AoMRC	Academy of Medical Royal Colleges
ARCP	Annual Review of Competence Progression
BMA	British Medical Association
BSc	Bachelor of Science
BSIR	British Society of Interventional Radiology
CASC	Clinical Assessment of Skills and Competencies
CAT	Core Anaesthesia Training
CCG	Clinical Commissioning Group
CCT	Certificate of Completion Training
CEGPR	Certificate of Eligibility for GP Registration
CESR	Certificate of Eligibility for Specialist Registration
COVID	'CO' stands for corona, 'VI' for virus, 'D' for disease.
CPD	Continuing Professional Development
CREST	Certificate of Readiness for Specialty Training
CrISP	Critically Ill Surgical Patient
CT	Computerised Tomography
CT2	Core trainee in the second year of training (CT1/CT3 etc)
CV	Curriculum Vitae
ED	Emergency department
EDAIC	European Diploma in Anaesthesiology and Intensive Care
ENT	Ear, Nose and Throat
EPIC	Electronic Portfolio of International Credentials
ERP	Emergency Registered Practitioner
FFICM	Fellowship of the Faculty of Intensive Care Medicine
FFOM	Fellowship of the Faculty of Occupational Medicine
FRCA	Fellowship of the Royal College of Anaesthetists
FRCEM	Fellowship of the Royal College of Emergency Medicine
FRCOphth	Fellowship of the Royal College of Ophthalmologists
FRCPath	Fellowship of the Royal College of Pathologists
FTE	Full-Time Equivalent
FY1	(or F1) Foundation Year 1
FY2	(or F2) Foundation year 2
FTE	Full-Time Equivalent (hours worked)
GMC	General Medical Council

GP	General Practice or General Practitioner
GPNRO	GP National Recruitment Office
GPST	General Practitioner Specialty Training
GROW	**G**oal, **R**eality, **O**ptions, **W**ay forward model
HEE	Health Education England
ICS	Integrated Care System
IELTS	International English Language Testing System
IMG	International Medical Graduate
IMT	Internal Medicine Training
JRCPTB	Joint Royal Colleges of Physicians Training Board
LAS	Locum Appointment for Service
LAT	Locum Appointment for Training
MCQ	Multiple Choice Question examination
MD	Doctor of Medicine
MFPH	Membership of the Faculty of Public Health
MPL	Medical Performers List
MRCGP	Member of the Royal College of General Practitioners
MRCOG	Member of the Royal College of Obstetricians and Gynaecologists
MRCP	Member of the Royal College of Physicians
MRCPCH	Member of the Royal College of Paediatrics and Child Health
MRCPsych	Member of the Royal College of Psychiatrists
MRCS	Member of the Royal College of Surgeons
MRI	Magnetic Resonance Imaging
MSRA	Multi-Specialty Recruitment Assessment
MTI	Medical Training Initiative
NASP	National Academy for Social Prescribing
NHS	National Health Service
NICE	National Institute for Health and Care Excellence
OCD	Obsessive Compulsive Disorder
OET	Occupational English Test
ORIEL	UK wide portal for recruitment to postgraduate medical, dental, public health, healthcare science and pre-registration pharmacy training
OSCE	Objective Structured Clinical Examination
PDSA	Plan, Do, Study, Act (cycles of audit)
PET	Positron Emission Tomography

PhD	Doctor of Philosophy
PRHO	Pre-registration House Officer (a term now replaced by Foundation Year)
PLAB	Professional Linguistics Assessments Board
PTSD	Post-Traumatic Stress Disorder
QI	Quality Improvement
RANRA	Rust Advanced Numerical Reasoning Appraisal
RCGP	Royal College of General Practitioners
RCOA	Royal College of Anaesthetists
RIS	Raw Interview Score
RCGP	Royal College of General Practitioners
RtP	Return to Practice
SAS	Specialty Doctors and Associate Specialists, or Staff Grade doctors
SOE	Structured Oral Examination
ST	Specialty Training
SWOT	Analysis of **S**trengths, **W**eaknesses, **O**pportunities and **T**hreats
TERS	Targeted Enhanced Recruitment Scheme
VUE	Virtual University Enterprises (now acquired by Pearson VUE for wide-ranging computer-based tests)
WHO	World Health Organisation
WTE	Whole Time Equivalent

Chapter 1. So many medical career paths – which/why/when/ how?

There are many career pathways and medical specialties in which doctors can choose to work in the UK. Before we start looking at the details of the range of medical specialty career pathways that a junior doctor could prioritise, or a doctor at any stage of their career could consider retraining for, let's consider the insights of two medical students about what their career ruminations and aspirations are, and the reflections of some experienced doctors too (you can learn more about their career progression on the www.mediroots.co.uk site where they each appear in videoed interviews).

Let's hear from Gabby Johnson, third year medical student, University of Nottingham:

Introduction

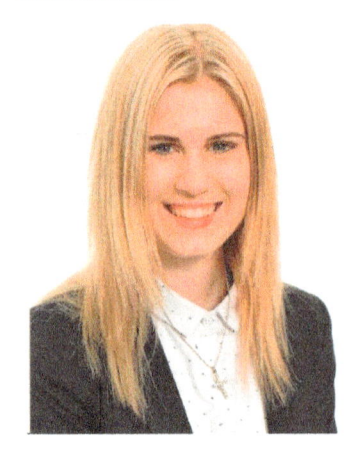

"I decided to do medicine as a young teenager because I always had a deep interest in science and also loved talking to people. I felt that medicine was the perfect combination between science, and helping and communicating with people of all different backgrounds and ages. I have a natural curiosity and passion to learn and I feel that a medical career will allow me to not only make a difference, but also to learn and develop as a person.

Medicine is a career that has a wide range of paths and avenues that can be explored and there are so many specialties to choose from. There are not many careers that have so many choices, that are so varied in nature but are as fulfilling and important as medicine is in the care of patients. I always loved the idea that medicine could be what I wanted it to be and that I can choose a career path that is right for me.

Insights as a medical student
Life as a medical student is so exciting and I am learning more every day in terms of knowledge and skills in relation to practising medicine, and also about myself. I am really enjoying my initial training and am looking forward to starting my first clinical placement soon. Progressing through medical school is of course not easy, but it is absolutely worth it. Currently at medical school I am commencing a dissertation in the area of immunology which will give me a great chance to delve into research - an element of medicine that I have not had much chance to explore yet. Medical school so far has been very varied and has given me the opportunity to learn about many areas of medicine to see what I enjoy the most and want to look into further, and consider which might be my future career paths. When commencing the clinical phase of my course I hope to have the chance to speak to many different physicians about their specialties and gain further insights.

So far in my quest to choosing a medical specialty I have been thinking about the areas that I have most interest in and several really intrigue me. Some of these options include genetics, haematology, oncology and many more. There are elements that I feel that I would prefer - such as working in a hospital setting - but I can't be completely sure until I go onto work in a clinical placement and experience it for myself to see what I do and don't like. That will give me many insights into different areas of medicine and what type of work I would like to be doing; this in turn will help me to choose my preferred specialty.

Choosing a specialty is something that I have been thinking about whilst I have been studying medicine in the last two years and there are not many career resources out there to help me to make that decision. Talking to various healthcare professionals in different roles will help me to gain insights into their specialties and what I would be doing on a day-to-day basis working in that area of medicine. It will help me to weigh up a number of factors such as my future work-life balance, to make sure that the specialty I choose is the right one for me long-term.

I think that MediRoots is a great medical careers resource as there are many videos of physicians from various different specialties giving their insights into their medical specialty and other allied roles and responsibilities that they have, by sharing and critiquing what they have done throughout their careers. I really like the way that each person discusses the things that they love about their specialty; but it is also really insightful to hear about the downsides so that I (and you) can make an informed careers decision after considering all aspects of their specialties. It is very useful to listen to an experienced doctor who has been working within their specialty for many years to allow me to gauge what my future career in that specialty could look like. It is really valuable to listen to people from specialties that you may not have considered before as it may be different to what you think and without MediRoots you may not get that opportunity to learn about that medical career pathway."

Finding meaning and letting your career choose you – Paul Beaney as a final year medical student shares his reflections:

Introduction

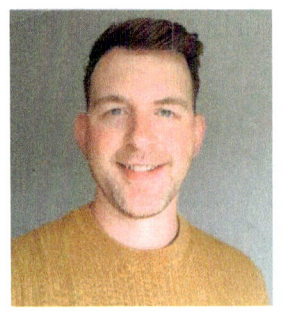

As a mature final year medical student who has just completed his second undergraduate degree, career options have never been far from my mind. Shortly after passing my final exams at the end of my fourth year, it became apparent to me that the long journey to become a qualified doctor since applying to medical school in 2014 (seven years ago) was nearly over. I often joke that before I decided to become a doctor the question I was always asked was 'So what do you want to do?' and that afterwards the question was 'So *now* what do you want do?' But that isn't the best question to ask. It's much better to ask: 'How can I live my life in a meaningful way so that I can fulfil my priorities for a worthwhile career and happy life in general?' But that isn't quite as snappy, so you can see why it hasn't caught on.

However, it's true. Rather than looking at choosing a career as a single decision, I have found it more useful to conceptualise it as a process of self-discovery and then the right path will choose me; if your medical career path hasn't become clear yet, then maybe you haven't asked yourself the right questions.

The best way I have found to ask those questions and learn the answers are to gain hands-on experience in frontline settings, talk to inspirational colleagues and perpetually self-reflect with a medical career in mind. Now I am still caught in limbo between conflicting interests and priorities, but I have made a lot of progress since I started on my medical journey.

Background

Before applying to medical school I had graduated with a Bachelor's degree in English and Philosophy five years earlier. I then worked in sales for four years and after never finding fulfilment I decided to embark on a totally new career path. To gain hands-on caring experience I became a full-time domiciliary care worker in my local community. After the initial culture shock, I knew that I had made the right choice and that healthcare was right for me. During this post I was confronted with the lack of resources in the social care setting and I was convinced that I should become a GP so that I could one day help to improve the community care situation. Six months later, I took my second job in healthcare as a theatre support worker in a busy Major Trauma Centre. I found the teamwork and practical skills required for surgery inspiring and it sparked a drive in me to become a surgeon. Seven years later and I am still torn between these two rather disparate career choices.

Foundation Programme

My present situation is that I have been accepted onto the Foundation Programme and became a newly qualified FY1 as of August 2021. I have decided to use this Foundation year to explore a variety of medical specialties that I have not had much experience in yet. Over the final year of my degree, I was exposed to specialties that I had ruled out of my career options, only to enjoy them and put them back on the list.
For example, as I was applying to the Foundation Programme, I was on a placement in the Emergency Department (ED). Prior to starting, I had ruled it out due to the preconceptions that I had about the challenging work-life balance in acute medical specialties. However, I found it thoroughly rewarding and despite the night shifts I enjoyed the diagnostic and decision-making elements of the job.

I took two things away from this experience: first, try different specialties before making too many assumptions about them. Second, it posed the question: which parts of medicine did I want to practise in? Do I want to make initial diagnoses and treat immediate issues? Or do I prefer making the definitive diagnosis and treating the patient through to discharge? It seems so obvious now but beforehand it had never really sunk in that different roles entail the use of various sets of skills (e.g. wound care versus pacemaker implantation) and knowledge (e.g. initial treatment versus long-term clinical management). Now whenever I consider an option, I try to find out what these are and whether that's what I would find satisfying.

Military Medicine
Aside from the NHS choices available to me, for the past 18 months I have been seriously exploring a career in military medicine. One of my concerns about this route was that post-F2 it would be three or four years before starting core/specialty training in the NHS, whilst completing my General Duties Medical Officer (GDMO) years in the Forces.
I attended an online 'acquaint' opportunity with the Royal Navy where I could talk directly to medical officers, other applicants and careers advisers. When I put this concern to the careers officer (also an ED consultant) he said that while it was true that my NHS career would be delayed, I would be a much better clinician than my peers when I did start training. He explained the high level of responsibility that you are given early on in the military field, forcing you to learn to make difficult decisions as you are often the only doctor on deployment. In contrast, in the NHS there is a lot more recourse to running things past a senior or another specialty doctor first. Furthermore, as an officer you are in a management role from day one, so you have a wealth of experience to draw on by the time you become a senior registrar/consultant, unlike most of your peers in the NHS. This advice resonated with me as it exposed areas within myself that I feel I need to develop in.
Ultimately for me, and after frank discussions with my partner, I concluded that despite all that a full-time naval career has to offer, at my stage of life (settling down and planning a family) the time I would spend on deployment in the years as a GDMO would be too great a sacrifice to make. However, I am not wholly deterred from this path as I am now exploring the option of joining the Royal Navy Reserves as a more flexible

way of combining family and military lives. Unless I had actively explored this option by attending the event and spoken to people with the relevant knowledge and experience, I wouldn't have reflected on and realised what my real priorities were i.e. being available for family life, and that I needed to improve my decision making and management skills going forward.

Conclusion

The experiences I had early on in frontline healthcare and medical school still exert a great influence on my overall career direction. But I have found that there are many other options still to consider. Life outside of medicine and the NHS is now influencing my career choices too. Despite still being in limbo between potential GP and surgery careers, I feel that I have come a long way in understanding myself, what I am suited to and what priorities I have outside of medicine - much better than before. My advice to anyone else is to be active in your decision-making process, talk to others and yourself as honestly as you can, take on experiences that interest you, reflect on them and consider your priorities both now and for the future. If my story says anything, it's that you can radically change career direction and find fulfilment where you least expected to; so long as you keep striving towards a meaningful life, the right career path will find you."

Hear how Dr Yazdan Zargham MBBS reached his decision to enter GP specialty training:

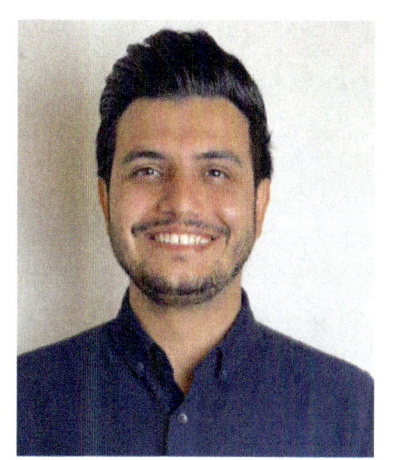

"Medicine has always been a passion of mine, requiring dedication, commitment and an ultimate drive for success. Growing up in a military family in Iran, my father instilled belief and hope in me for achieving my goals. This is something that is intrinsic to my outlook on life and medical practice; and still strongly embedded in my everyday life. This belief and encouragement led me to study medicine.

I started medicine at 17-years old in Armenia, where I then lived and worked for seven years. Studying in a foreign country allowed me to integrate with different cultures and lifestyles, yet provided me with the medical knowledge and skills necessary to practise as a doctor upon graduation.

After finishing my medical degree, I returned to Iran, to gain further experience and better my career prospects; although, this did not go to plan as I had to leave my country. Upon arriving in the UK in 2015, I did not know whether I would be able to practise medicine again. Whilst applying for my leave to remain, I volunteered at a local church, serving the homeless with meals, cleaning and maintaining the daily running of the church, and at times, translating for other Iranians who did not speak English. It was at the church that I met two nurses, Susie and Jayne, who both took an interest in my background as a doctor. This changed my life. The nurses introduced me to Professor Ruth Chambers who had been supporting local refugee doctors, and therefore helped me to practise again in the UK.

During this time, I have had to sit a number of English and medical exams including IELTS and both PLAB exams. This progressed as I completed the GMC's requirements and then the UK Foundation Programme, which I undertook at the University Hospital of North Midlands and the University Hospitals of Derby and Burton NHS Foundation Trust.
My rotations included Chemical Pathology, General Surgery, Palliative Care, Acute Medicine and Trauma and Orthopaedics. This enabled me to consolidate my knowledge and skills, as well as learn about the English healthcare system which I am now an integral part of.

Since starting as a junior doctor, with the varied training path completed as part of my Foundation Programme, I contemplated the direction of my career path in terms of my future medical specialty choices. After careful and informed speculation, I decided on GP specialty training, due to the benefits that I perceived that this career path offers in terms of business opportunities, a more flexible lifestyle, as well as the potential to develop a special interest with hands on practice at the NHS frontline.

Having only just started my GP specialty training pathway, I hope to use each opportunity I have to not only enhance my own medical career, but also to help to inform the choice of career pathways for other junior doctors and medical students. I have enjoyed writing this book conveying career insights of a number of medical speciality training pathways and have developed a website www.mediroots.co.uk, where I have collated interviews with senior consultants and medical students about their experiences in their choice of medical specialty. I hope I am able to split my time between medical practice, and educating the prospective future medical workforce in the UK."

The exciting career path of Professor Helen Stokes Lampard FRCGP, PhD, FLSW:

Helen is a GP Principal, Chair of the Academy of Medical Royal Colleges (AoMRC), the umbrella body for all Royal Colleges and Faculties in the UK, Chair of the Board of the National Academy for Social Prescribing (NASP) and Professor of GP Education. She was Chair of the Royal College of General Practitioners (RCGP) until November 2019.

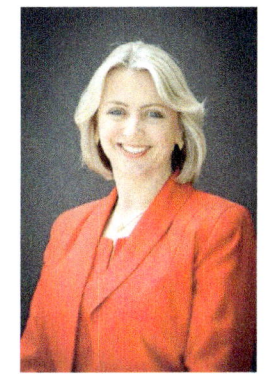

Helen went to medical school intending to specialise in gynaecological oncology and found that she enjoyed every clinical specialty that she encountered. As a junior doctor, she changed her career direction and took up academic general practice – difficult at the time but "The most wonderful swerve of my life in terms of career, fulfilment and opportunities." Prior to training as a GP, she had worked in Obstetrics and Gynaecology for several years and this experience shaped her clinical and academic aspirations.

She began working at the University of Birmingham's Department of Primary Care in 2000, while she was a GP registrar. She gained a PhD in 2009; the subject being 'Variation in NHS utilisation of vault cytology tests in women post-hysterectomy'. Her diverse research interests have spanned gynaecological cancer screening, all aspects of women's health, epidemiology and data linkage studies.

Helen had various academic roles including a stint as Head of Primary Care (undergraduate) in the Medical School of the University of Birmingham, Clinical Director of a Trials unit and Head of GP Education prior to becoming the Chair of the RCGP. She was also a trained personal mentor for 'doctors in difficulty' in the Midlands until 2016; a scheme supported by the West Midlands Deanery and RCGP Midlands Faculty.

During her time as RCGP Chair, Helen had a high media profile with over 200 TV, 200 radio and 20,000 appearances in printed media (newspapers) and she led several major professional gains; including state backed indemnity for all NHS staff working in the community, a new vision for General Practice and implementation of significant financial and contractual improvements in GPs' working lives.

As Chair of AoMRC she sits on numerous national committees including the National Escalation Pressures Panel, the review of digital healthcare and the NHS Net Zero Executive, as well as a large number focussed on urgent reshaping of the NHS in response to the COVID-19 pandemic. She is fully seconded away from the University of Birmingham for the duration of this role (2020-23).

As Chair of the Board of NASP, she is helping to shape their direction, building strong partnerships, establishing an academic basis for the social prescribing movement and raising its profile. Helen remains a part-time GP partner at The Westgate Practice in Lichfield, Staffordshire.

She is naturally enthusiastic and dynamic with a sense of humour and plenty of pragmatism.

Insights from the 50 years medical career path of Professor Ruth Chambers OBE, MD, FRCGP:

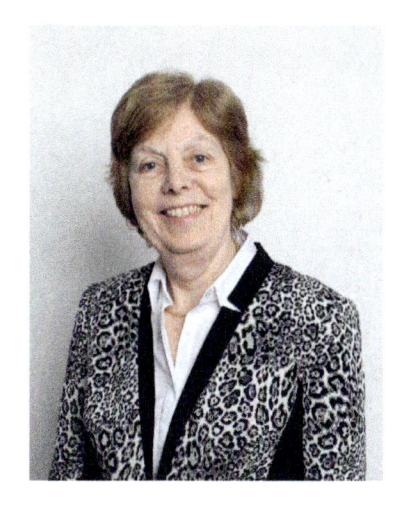

"I first contemplated being a doctor in my last year of secondary school when a friend picked medicine in her University application form – and I thought 'If Sarah can apply then I will too.' I hedged my bets by also applying for pharmacy, and then agriculture college if my A level grades were really low. And in those days most medical schools had a 10% limit on the recruitment of female medical students. My A levels were good enough for Nottingham University Medical School (1970) and I absorbed their community health care ethos, where unusually in those days community doctors and GPs were seen as valued doctors, and not necessarily on the career paths for a doctor who was unsuccessful in entering hospital medical specialties.

As I worked as a junior doctor in hospital I became aware of the 'control freak' nature of hospital bosses to hospital medical consultants. I thought it would be boring to have a narrow specialty where I provided the 'same old/same old' medical care week after week and so I opted for general practice where I thought I could be more my own boss and have a diverse medical career with a wide spectrum of patients and health conditions. That led to three year GP specialty training in Bristol (which was not essential training to be a GP in those days, just an option), alongside which I had two children for whom my husband paused his career to be the house-parent whilst I worked long medic shifts. I moved to a salaried GP post for three years (where I learnt first hand about prescription fraud – then shared those insights in a lead role with the Department of Health some years later, leading to the national NHS fraud system being established).

Then I shifted to a GP partnership in Stone, Staffordshire for 10 years, where I developed my research interest alongside, undertaking a master's degree that converted to a doctorate over 8 academic years, focused on doctors' health. This led to my leading a national Department of Health funded programme too on combating doctors' stress, in association with the Royal College of GPs.

Since then I have had many fixed-term national roles with the NHS, Royal Colleges, Charities, NICE and others, alongside my GP career, always with a focus on sharing the learning – in publications, at conferences (across the UK and the world e.g. USA, Canada, Tunisia, European countries, Hong Kong, Japan and more) and moved from being an employed University professor at Staffordshire University, to honorary posts at Staffordshire and Keele Universities. With this interest in medical education, I became Director of Postgraduate training across the West Midlands for GP, nursing and other primary care specialties in 2006 for a few years.

I've expanded my interests and roles to designing and leading on funded quality improvement programmes at scale – mainly focused on primary care (for which I got an OBE in 2013) but also other NHS organisations and social care, with an underpinning thread of patient self-care and empowerment. Until recently I was Clinical Chair of Stoke-on-Trent Clinical Commissioning Group (CCG) and I retired as a practising GP after 40+ years. For the last three years I have focused on disseminating technology enabled care in the NHS, digital upskilling of clinicians and social workers and social prescribers and improving digital literacy of local patients (including support for refugees and asylum seekers), developing apps with a co-design approach, deploying personal digital assistants such as Alexa Echo Shows to those in need for their health & wellbeing, with external funds.

Over my career I have written 76 books (yes 76!!) – mainly for health care teams, some for the public on health conditions such as back pain/healthy heart/work stress, and more recent ones on digital transformation of health and self-care from clinicians' and patients' perspectives; and written many health articles in medical magazines and my local newspaper."

Mediroots & branches of successful medical careers

The tree below captures the key themes that have emerged from the interviews with the many experienced doctors captured on the MediRoots website and relays their 'routes' to successful career pathways.

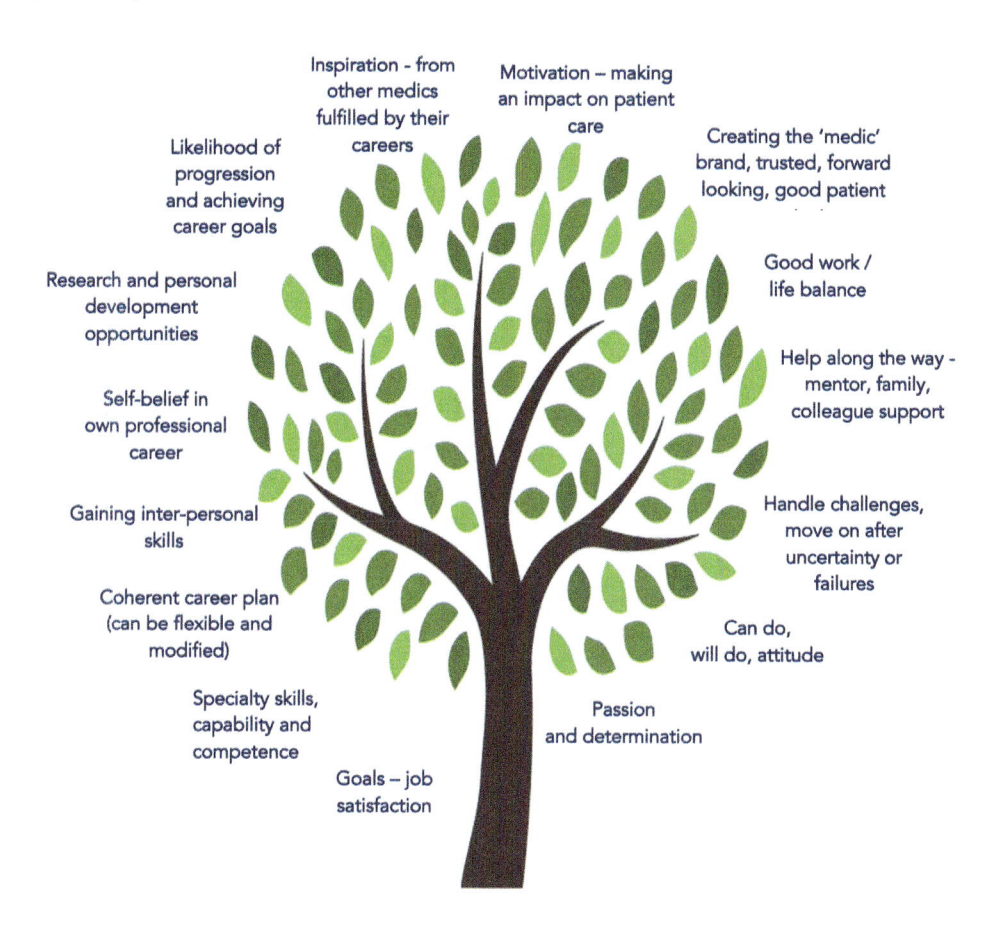

Inspiration - from other medics fulfilled by their careers

Motivation – making an impact on patient care

Creating the 'medic' brand, trusted, forward looking, good patient

Likelihood of progression and achieving career goals

Good work / life balance

Research and personal development opportunities

Help along the way - mentor, family, colleague support

Self-belief in own professional career

Handle challenges, move on after uncertainty or failures

Gaining inter-personal skills

Coherent career plan (can be flexible and modified)

Can do, will do, attitude

Specialty skills, capability and competence

Passion and determination

Goals – job satisfaction

Mediroots & branches of successful medical careers

Chapter 2. The UK context for medical specialty training of junior doctors

The medical workforce in the UK

Many health professionals undergo multiple transitions during their career pathways. Yet there is little known about the sources of careers information they access and limited availability of good careers guidance, support and advice services. So doctors and other health professionals may end up in posts to which they are ill suited. They may have pursued different career pathways if only appropriate careers advice had been readily available earlier on, and throughout their careers. And for many, their career objectives and career progress is central to their personal morale and job satisfaction.

The British Medical Association (BMA) is very vocal that we are not training enough doctors in the UK.[1] Demand is soaring with the huge backlog of care post–pandemic, the increasing numbers of people aged 85 years and over (nearly doubling from 1.6 million in 2018 to an expected three million by 2043) and the overall growth of the population. In total the NHS in England employs 159,100 full-time equivalent (FTE) doctors, including all grades of secondary care doctors and general practitioners. England has a relatively low doctor to population ratio of 2.8 doctors per 1000 population compared to most European countries; and this ratio is becoming worse as the population expands and the medical workforce reduces so that there are just 0.46 fully qualified GPs per 1000 patients in England in 2021, down from 0.52 in 2015. The number of FTE doctors working in secondary care in 2021 was 18.5% more in 2021 compared with 2015, on the other hand. Some specialties have shrunk - for instance the numbers of occupational medicine consultant posts fell by 34% in 2021 compared with 2009; and some have more posts per specialty in different regions of England – for instance there are proportionately more geriatric medicine posts in London despite there being the lowest proportion of over-65 year olds living in London compared with the rest of the country. The distribution of NHS doctors across the country is currently not proportionate to the population in each region; for instance there are 3.5million more people residing in the Midlands compared to the North West of England, who have access to 4,000 fewer hospital based doctors. The BMA has calculated that we need to scale up our medical workforce by an additional 31% to bring the total FTE count to 208,262 FTE doctors for England to be equivalent to other comparator European countries – which equates to a current medical workforce deficit of 49,162 FTE doctors. To add to this, the medical workforce is ageing, with 13% of secondary care doctors and 18% of GPs due to reach minimum retirement age (55 years old) within the next ten years.[2,3]

The NHS medical training and practice structure

This can be confusing when you are new to it and a relative outsider as a medical student - even for Foundation doctors. So in essence the structure of career progression is:

Undergraduate Medical Students: in the UK, medical students typically study for five years with much of their last three years spent in teaching hospitals and teaching general practices.

Foundation Doctors: graduates from medical school enter their two-year Foundation Training Programme with a sequence of six x four months posts in a varied range of specialties of medicine and surgery. Doctors in the Foundation Year One (FY1) programme are provisionally registered with the General Medical Council (GMC); and when they successfully finish their FY1 year are then fully registered with a licence to practise by the GMC as Foundation Year Two (FY2) doctors. This allows them to take on more responsibility for providing patient care - under the supervision of experienced doctors and other healthcare professionals.

It is possible to take a break between Foundation and Specialty training, via a Foundation Year 3 post. This might help the doctor get more experience of specialties they've not yet tried in their first two years of Foundation training, and explore different avenues, enabling them to define and reinforce their career goals. Such a FY3 year can help the doctor to strengthen their portfolio ready for future specialty applications, especially if their preferred specialty is highly sought after with a competitive entry rate (see Table 3.1); or they have experienced the way that some individuals (e.g. senior doctors and medical school staff) stereotype some specialties and indulge in sarcastic remarks and banter that disrespects other colleagues and their clinical focus.

Core Training Doctors: Core Surgical training, Acute Care Common Stem (ACCS) and Internal Medicine Training (IMT) and some other medical specialties require doctors to have undertaken a more generic programme of training before entering specialty training. Doctors can then apply for higher specialty training in a specific medical specialty area after completing these training programmes.

Specialty Training (ST) Doctors: doctors enrolled on a specialty training programme may have previously completed a core training programme before entering higher specialist training; or for some specialties such as general practice, they will have progressed into specialty training after completing their FY2 programme. Specialty training programmes take between three to eight years to complete depending on the nature of the specialty, with progressively less supervision from experienced doctors and other healthcare professionals in their final year(s).

Consultants and General Practitioners: upon completing their specialty training and related final examinations, doctors gain a Certificate of Completion Training (CCT). This allows them to apply to the relevant Trust or employer for a post in their chosen specialty, or to a GP practice or related employer to become a consultant or general practitioner, amending their personal details on the GMC register in line with their licence to practise.

Specialty Doctors and Associate Specialists (SAS): SAS doctors include staff grade, associate specialist and specialty doctors with at least four years of postgraduate training, where at least two of which are in a relevant specialty.

Locally Employed or Salaried Doctors: some doctors opt to work in non-training roles such as in a Trust grade post, as a clinical fellow, or being directly employed by a Trust or general practice for relevant service posts.

Flexible working: over the years the NHS has developed retention schemes and ways to adapt jobs to match the needs or preferences of individual doctors. Some Trusts and other NHS employers offer flexible working opportunities to try to boost recruitment, retention, motivation and employee productivity. These might be by shift swapping, annualised hours, part-time working, job-sharing, a regular day off to compensate for hours worked outside normal working hours. Flexible working practices allow for doctors to develop portfolio careers that include balancing clinical, managerial or academic work with two or more part-time posts by different employers (e.g. a Trust and a University), or incorporating different responsibilities as a Trust might do for a Medical Director who still practises at the frontline in their medical specialty, or has a clinical lead position in the local integrated care system engaging with others across the local health and care system.

Supervision
As a doctor in training you are assigned a clinical supervisor for each four months placement, who is usually a consultant working in the same department as you and can provide supervision for the clinical work you undertake in your post. Your educational supervisor will help you to develop a personal development plan and will oversee your education and professional development for some time throughout your Foundation training, or even for the whole of your training programme.

You should book regular discussions with your supervisors reviewing your progress and outstanding educational needs. These discussions should also include an oversight and reflection of your strengths and weaknesses in your clinical post(s); evidence of your achievements and any difficulties you are experiencing such as significant events and complaints.

As a doctor in training, you will be required to complete a portfolio; typically an electronic portfolio, or e-portfolio. Every training programme or medical specialty will have a slightly different e-portfolio matched to the differing curriculum requirements that is expected to be completed by their trainees.

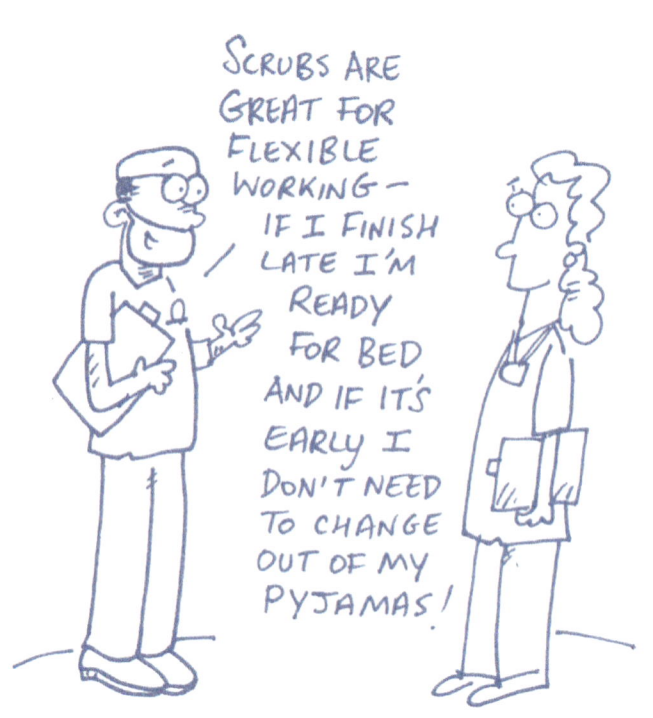

References

1. British Medical Association (BMA). Medical staffing in England: a defining moment for doctors and patients. London: BMA. July 2021.
https://www.bma.org.uk/media/4316/bma-medical-staffing-report-in-england-july-2021.pdf

2. NHS Digital. NHS Workforce Statistics. London: NHS Digital. February 2021. https://digital.nhs.uk/data-and-information/publications/statistical/nhs-workforce-statistics/december-2020

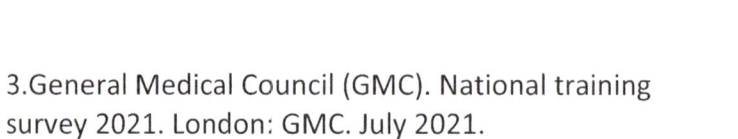

3. General Medical Council (GMC). National training survey 2021. London: GMC. July 2021.
https://www.gmc-uk.org/-/media/documents/national-training-survey-results-2021---summary-report_pdf-87050829.pdf

Chapter 3. Get familiar with the range of medical specialty training pathways

Medical Career Pathways

There are so many medical specialties with varying training requirements and programmes. Then there are sub-specialties, with extended roles such as in teaching or management, academic and research posts, differing health care settings such as urban or rural practice and types of hospitals or general practices.

The services provided by the NHS are organised into the following categories:

Primary care includes community services such as general practice, general dentistry, pharmacies, walk-in clinics, the NHS 111 telephone service and community optometry. It is usually the first point of contact for patients and a route to access secondary care services.

Secondary care is healthcare generally provided in hospitals, which includes accident and emergency departments, inpatient wards, outpatient departments, antenatal services, mental health hospitals and sexual health clinics.

Tertiary care is the services provided for people needing complex treatments. Patients may be referred for tertiary care (for example, a specialist stroke unit) by either primary care or secondary care health professionals.

With all this complexity, many medical students or doctors need help in actively selecting and managing their career paths. They will require information and intelligence about the variety of medical careers available and how to access them. Or they may require more individualised help, identifying the factors that are important to them in selecting a discipline or new specialist area and picturing their priorities in terms of skills, interests and what motivates them.

Doctors in established careers also may want to reassess their career to date or explore new opportunities (even retrain in a different medical specialty), or address gaps in their current knowledge or skills or experience.

Table 3.1 captures the numbers of doctors applying to specific medical specialty training posts in England, the numbers accepted and percentage of training posts filled – for the 2019 and 2021.

You'll see in the latest data, that there were 3733 available posts for GP specialty training with a 98.9% fill rate…ranging to only five available posts for cardiothoracic surgery specialty training with a 100% fill rate![1]

You can also find out more about career options for doctors available in the UK on the https://www.healthcareers.nhs.uk/explore-roles/doctors site.

Or for specific advice on general practice careers take a look at the GP Careers Hub on the NHS Futures platform: https://future.nhs.uk/GPCS/groupHome

Table 3.1 Medical specialty recruitment update for 2021 compared to 2019: posts, acceptance and fill rates[1]

Training Programme	2021 Posts	2021 Accepts	2021 Fill Rate %	2019 Posts	2019 Accepts	2019 Fill Rate %
Internal Medicine Training	1313	1313	100.0%	1364	1357	99.5%
Anaesthetics	450	450	100.0%	450	450	100.0%
Emergency Medicine	320	320	100.0%	331	324	97.9%
Cardio-thoracic surgery	5	5	100.0%	10	10	100.0%
Clinical Radiology	300	300	100.0%	250	249	99.6%
Community Sexual and Reproductive Health	5	5	100.0%	5	5	100.0%
Core Psychiatry Training	428	425	99.3%	412	381	92.5%
Core Surgical Training	495	476	96.2%	515	515	100.0%
General Practice	3733	3690	98.9%	3250	2981	91.7%
Histopathology	89	89	100.0%	76	76	100.0%
Neurosurgery	13	13	100.0%	21	21	100.0%
Obstetrics and Gynaecology	226	226	100.0%	231	223	96.5%
Ophthalmology	76	76	100.0%	79	79	100.0%
Oral and Maxillo-facial surgery	10	10	100.0%	6	6	100.0%
Paediatrics	368	368	100.0%	419	347	82.8%
Public Health Medicine	80	80	100.0%	77	77	100.0%
Total	7911	7846	99.2%	7496	7101	94.7%

[1] Health Education England.
Medical specialty recruitment update 2019-2021: posts, acceptance and fill rates
https://www.hee.nhs.uk/our-work/medical-recruitment/specialty-recruitment-round-1-acceptance-fill-rate

(data accessed 30.8.21 from http://www.oriel.nhs.uk)

Medical specialty entry requirement and training pathways

Here is an overview of a wide range of ten medical specialties – what each specialty post entails, the application process and routes along the training pathways.

1. ANAESTHETICS

What is an anaesthetist?
Anaesthetists are specialist doctors who are responsible for providing anaesthesia to patients for operations and procedures. Their range of practice may extend beyond anaesthesia; for example pain management and intensive care.
Anaesthetists form the largest specialty group of doctors in NHS hospitals. Their postgraduate specialist training spans at least seven years in anaesthesia, intensive care medicine and pain management. Most consultant anaesthetists develop subspecialist interests in a particular area of surgical practice, or in pain management or critical care, or educational roles including supervision of junior doctors in training.

What does an anaesthetist do?
An anaesthetist meets with the patient and surgical team in order to plan what sort of anaesthetic is most appropriate. This may be on the day of the surgery for straightforward operations, or in an anaesthetic pre-assessment clinic for those patients who will require more complex surgery. Routine checks and preparations are then made for the specific patients on that day's operating list.

In theatre, the anaesthetist tailors the anaesthetic delivered to the individual patient and remains with them throughout the operation, monitoring and treating them as necessary for the effects of the anaesthetic and the scope of the surgery and how it progresses. This may include simple monitoring of the heart, blood pressure and oxygen levels, right through to provision of advanced organ support in complex cases. Anaesthetists also plan and implement pain relief to ensure that patients are comfortable immediately following their operation.

After the operation or procedure, the anaesthetist is responsible for the patient in the recovery area until the effects of the anaesthetic have worn off enough for the patient to return to their hospital ward. Where complex types of pain relief are used on the ward the anaesthetists in the pain service team may provide follow on care and continue to review these patients until their need for pain relief is over.

Other roles in anaesthetics

All trainee anaesthetists undergo specialist training in intensive care medicine. Most of the consultants in intensive care medicine and associated resuscitation teams are anaesthetists, and are often involved in training other clinicians too.

Anaesthetics is a diverse specialty. Anaesthetists who specialise in pain management may focus on pain in childbirth and patients with long-term or chronic pain problems, as well as adult patients with chronic pain problems. Other areas anaesthetists might specialise in include: imaging, scanning, endoscopy, dental treatment.

Entry requirements for anaesthetics

Dr Yazdan has extracted interesting information from the useful sources listed below, to guide you the reader as to the entry requirements and application process for this medical specialty.

See these **Useful sources:**
1. Royal College of Anaesthetists – Self-Assessment Criteria:

https://anro.wm.hee.nhs.uk/Portals/3/Documents/National/Self-Assessment%20Criteria%20AnaestheticsACCS%20Anaesthetics%20CT1(2020).pdf?ver=2019-10-21-090856-733

2. Anaesthesia (Person Specification):
https://specialtytraining.hee.nhs.uk/portals/1/Content/Person%20Specifications/Anaesthesia/ANAESTHESIA%20-%20CT1%202021.pdf

3. Royal College of Anaesthetists:
https://www.rcoa.ac.uk

Entry requirements for Anaesthetics Specialty training include:

Essential
1. Completion of a medical degree 2. Completion of the UK Foundation Programme 3. A PASS in the Multi-Specialty Recruitment Assessment 4. Portfolio of competencies 5. Interview
Desirable
• Experience of 18 months or less in anaesthetics (not including Foundation training modules) by time of intended start date • Ability to use your judgement and make decisions • Knowledge of medicine • Ability to work well with your hands • Thinking and reasoning skills • To be thorough and pay attention to detail • Excellent verbal communication skills • Ability to accept criticism and work well under pressure • Patience and the ability to remain calm in stressful situations • Ability to use a computer and the main software packages competently

The Person Specification is one of the most important documents for Anaesthetics Recruitment, as it outlines the requirements for entry onto the training programme. It includes the following domains:
1. Commitment to anaesthetics (attendance at courses/taster week/observation)
2. Qualifications – including BSc, MD, PhD and postgraduate qualifications e.g. MRCP, MRCS
3. Research – particularly anaesthetics related
4. Audit – completion of an anaesthetics related audit
5. Teaching – teaching of colleagues/medical students etc.
6. Management and Leadership – examples of leadership and management/management related courses completed

The portfolio should be mapped against the person specification in order to achieve the highest-ranking scores.

Structure of anaesthetics training
There are four levels of anaesthestics training:
1. Basic or Core Level (2-3 years)
2. Intermediate Level (2 years)
3. Higher Level (2 years)
4. Advanced Level (1 year)

This forms the entire training programme to Certificate of Completion of Training (CCT), which takes around 7-8 years. The extra one year depends on the route of entry to the training. Anaesthetics training is not a run-through programme. Two recruitment phases take place at the basic/core level (ST1) and the intermediate level (ST3).

Basic or core level (CT1-2 OR ACCS)
Before applying for this level, you must demonstrate these three things:
1. Full GMC registration
2. Foundation Competencies (CREST)
3. Less then 18 months of total clinical work experience in anaesthetics.

If you meet the entry criteria, there are two routes of entry:
1. Core Anaesthesia Training (CAT) (2 Years)
2. Acute Care Common Stem (ACCS) (3 Years)

What is ACCS?
ACCS is a three year alternative core training programme to enter specialty training in General Internal Medicine, Acute Internal Medicine or Anaesthetics, and is the main core training module for Emergency Medicine. The first two years are spent rotating through Emergency Medicine, General Internal Medicine, Anaesthetics and Intensive Care Medicine. The last year is to ensure that all requirements are met for entry into your chosen specialty.

Gaining Fellowship of Royal College of Anaesthetics (FRCA)

Primary FRCA must be passed on entry to ST3 to be considered eligible. This exam has two parts (taken separately):
1. Multiple Choice Question Examination (MCQ)
2. The Objective Structured Clinical Examination (OSCE) and Structured Oral Examination (SOE)

The final FRCA must be completed prior to Higher and Advanced Level Training.

Intermediate level (ST3-4)

The Intermediate level spans two years and introduces trainees to specialist areas of anaesthesia. Eligibility is dependent on:
1. Full GMC registration
2. Primary FRCA or having an exempting qualification
3. Evidence of achievement of CT2 competences in Anaesthetics and Intensive Care Medicine
4. At least 24 months experience in Anaesthetics and/or Intensive Care Medicine

Higher and advanced level (ST5-6-7)

To enter into the higher and advanced level, an intermediate level trainee must pass the final FRCA exam. The higher level training is two years in duration and is termed post-fellowship training. On completion of this, a trainee will be considered to have become a specialist and receive their CCT.

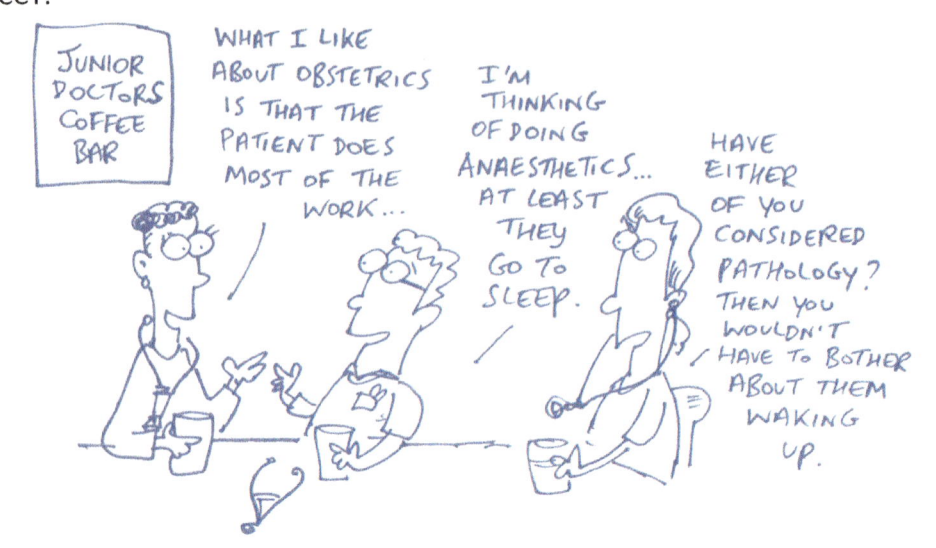

2. CLINICAL RADIOLOGY

What is radiology?
Radiology is a medical specialty, focusing on imaging to diagnose and treat diseases seen in the body. Imaging may include:
- X-Ray
- Ultrasound
- Computed Tomography (CT)
- Nuclear medicine including Positron Emission Tomography (PET) and Magnetic Resonance Imaging (MRI).

Interventional radiology is the performance of medical procedures with the guidance of imaging technology. These procedures are usually minimally invasive. There are many interventional techniques including:
- Oesophageal stents
- Angioplasty
- Angiography
- Biliary drainage and stenting
- Needle biopsy
- Treatment of internal bleeding
- Treatment of arteriovenous malformations.

Interventional radiology is defined as a sub-specialty, recognised by the GMC. Other areas of special interest include: breast, cardiac, emergency, gastrointestinal, head and neck, interventional, musculoskeletal, neuroradiology, oncology, paediatric, radionuclide, thoracic, uro-gynaecological, vascular.

What is a radiologist?
A radiologist is a specialty trained doctor who interprets imaging to guide the management of diseases. Radiologists work closely with radiographers who perform the imaging; and they work closely with the multi-disciplinary team, to provide insightful expert reports that guide the correct management and treatment of patients requiring radiology. An interventional radiologist will perform a procedure, such as an angiogram or a biopsy under imaging technology.

Entry requirements for radiology

Dr Yazdan has extracted interesting information from the useful sources listed below, to guide you the reader as to the entry requirements and application process for this medical specialty.

See these **Useful sources:**

Royal College of Radiologists – https://www.rcr.ac.uk/

British Medical Association - https://www.bma.org.uk/

British Society of Interventional Radiology - https://www.bsir.org/

The entry requirements for Radiology Specialty training include:

Essential
1. Completion of a medical degree
2. Completion of the UK Foundation Programme
3. A PASS in the Multi-Specialty Recruitment Assessment
4. Portfolio
5. Interview
Desirable
Clinical radiologists need: <ul><li>An analytical mind, an eye for detail and good observational skills</li><li>Keen interest in anatomy, physiology and pathology</li><li>Good understanding of general medicine and surgery</li><li>Manual dexterity for certain roles</li><li>Good clinical knowledge across all specialties</li><li>Good organisational ability and ability to manage a busy role</li><li>Ability to work well in a team and to manage others effectively</li><li>Excellent verbal communication skills to deal with patients and colleagues</li><li>Excellent written communication skills for accurate report-writing.</li></ul>

The Person Specification is one of the most important documents for Clinical Radiology Recruitment, as it outlines the requirements for entry on to a Radiology Specialty Training Programme.

It includes the following domains:

1. Commitment to Radiology (attendance at courses/taster week/observation)
2. Qualifications – including BSc, MD, PhD and post-graduate exams e.g. MRCP, MRCS
3. Research – particular radiology related
4. Audit – Completion of a radiology related audit
5. Teaching – teaching of colleagues/medical students etc.
6. Management and Leadership – examples of leadership and management/management related courses.

A good tip is that the trainee's portfolio content should be mapped against the person specification in order to achieve the highest ranking scores in the specialty application process.

Clinical radiology application process

1. ORIEL

Applications are made through the ORIEL online portal, a national application process throughout England, Scotland Wales, & Northern Ireland. The ORIEL application form contains a self-assessment score, which is based on the candidate's personal achievements. All evidence to support this should be uploaded on the ORIEL platform. This portfolio self-assessment score is verified by radiology consultants.

2. Preferencing

Once applying for Clinical Radiology specialty training, you will be asked to rank regions in order of preferences. It is important you only rank areas where you will be willing to work. For example, no. 1 is considered most preferred, no.2 is your next most wanted etc. If you do not wish to work in a particular area, you must indicate 'not wanted'.

3. Completion of the multi-specialty recruitment assessment (MSRA)

All candidates are required to PASS the MSRA exam. This exam consists of two papers:
1. Professional Dilemma Paper
2. Clinical Problem-Solving Paper

The Professional Dilemma Paper is similar to a situational judgement examination and requires individuals to think about how to act as a doctor in particular situations. More specifically, it requires candidates to demonstrate integrity, coping under pressure, sensitivity, empathy and recognising and prioritising workload.

The Clinical Problem-Solving Paper – assesses 12 different subject areas (Cardiovascular, Dermatology/ENT/Ophthalmology, Endocrine/Metabolic, Gastroenterology/Nutrition, Infectious Diseases/Haematology/Immunology/Allergies/Genetics, Musculoskeletal, Paediatrics, Pharmacology, Psychiatry/Neurology, Renal/Urology, Reproductive/Obstetrics and Gynaecology, Respiratory).

Questions are focused on investigations, diagnosis, emergencies, prescribing and management.

4. Ranking

Ranking is based on the:
1. MSRA Score
2. Portfolio Self-Assessment Score
3. Interview Score

The application process was devised in its current form in 2016, using the MSRA to shortlist candidates. From 2020, not all candidates have needed to be interviewed. The top 55 ranking candidates bypass the interview stage based on their MSRA score and portfolio self-assessment score. The remaining candidates are interviewed - usually virtually.

5. Virtual interviews

The interview consists of three stations:
1. Preparation station – requiring the candidate to score their portfolio against a pre-determined mark sheet.
2. Verification of the portfolio – screening of portfolio with examiners, followed by a brief discussion.
3. Commitment to Radiology station – general themed station to demonstrate the candidate's understanding of the specialty and capture their reasons for choosing Clinical Radiology.

The candidate's interview score is added to their MSRA and portfolio self-assessment scores.

6. Offers

Candidates are ranked according to their overall score and offers are made based on their overall score and ranking preferences.

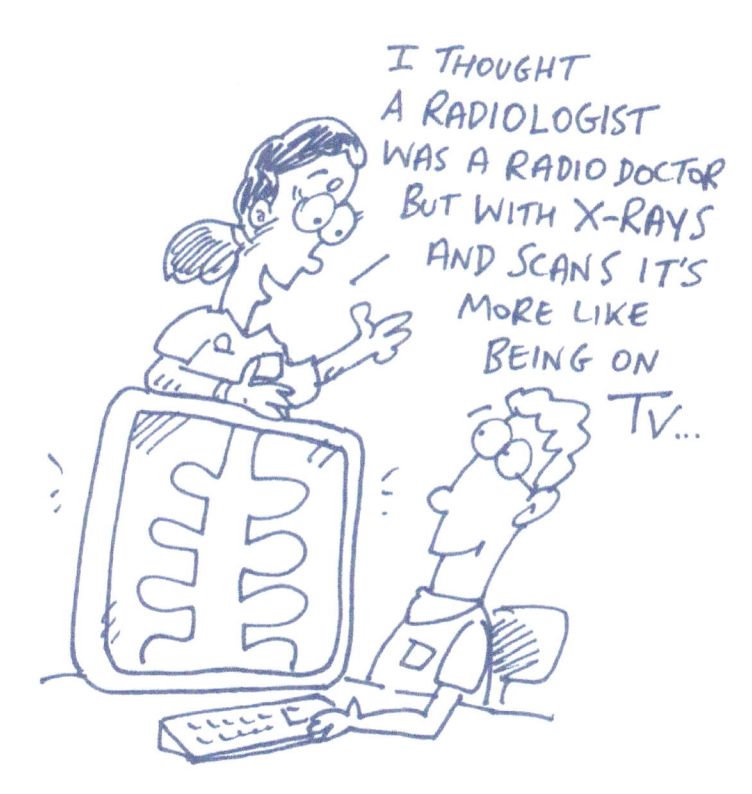

3. GENERAL PRACTICE

What is a general practitioner?
The Royal College of General Practitioners (RCGP), the British Medical Association (BMA) and General Medical Council (GMC) recognise that GPs are expert medical generalists, and as such are specialists in general practice. General practitioners are expected to work in a variety of primary care settings and are considered to be the first point of contact for patients. This role encompasses a wide range of clinical skills and knowledge, due to the variety of services offered within primary care settings.

In 2007, the current GP Specialty Training was formally introduced in the UK, replacing previous models of training. This followed the revision of the criteria within the regulatory framework of the Postgraduate Medical Education and Training Board for approval of specialist training in general practice. Since 2006 the 'GP Register' has been in place to provide assurance to patients, employers and the profession that a doctor has achieved the standards, knowledge and skills required to practise safely at a senior level.

Entry requirements for GP Specialty Training
Dr Yazdan has extracted interesting information from the useful sources listed below, to guide you the reader as to the entry requirements and application process for this medical specialty.

See these **Useful sources:**
1. Oriel Applicant User Guide (for general guidance on how to navigate Oriel and technical help with the on-line application form).

2. 2021 Medical Specialty Recruitment Applicant Handbook (for general information about the administration of national recruitment processes).

3. GPNRO website (for dates and deadlines for the next set of applications).

Essential
1. Completion of a medical degree
2. Completion of the UK Foundation Programme
3. PASS in the MSRA examination
Desirable
- Ability to listen and communicate effectively
- Strong interest in working with people
- Ability to work in a multi-disciplinary team
- Willingness and ability to handle uncertainty and conflicting demands
- Ability to stay calm while working under pressure
- Excellent organisational and time-management skills
- Entrepreneurial and business skills, or willingness to develop these if you decide to become a GP partner
- Good IT skills
- Ability to manage change

The GP application process

1. **ORIEL**

All applications are made electronically via the ORIEL recruitment portal website. You will be asked to provide factual information about you and your employment history. There is a two-week window to apply via ORIEL, after which you will hear if you have been invited to attend the MRSA exam or interview. This is communicated via email.

2. **Preferencing**

You will be asked to rank regions in order of preferences. It is important you only rank areas which you will be willing to work in. For example, no. 1 is considered to be your preferred choice, no.2 is your next most wanted etc. If you do not wish to work in a particular area, you must indicate 'not wanted'. Choosing preferences takes careful consideration, as GP specialty training is a three year programme, and may determine where you practise in the future.

The Targeted Enhanced Recruitment Scheme (TERS) is a national incentive scheme which offers a one-off payment of £20,000 (pre-tax) for accepting a GP post in an area which has been difficult to recruit to for the past three years.

3. Multi-specialty recruitment assessment (MSRA)

All candidates are required to PASS the MSRA exam. This exam consists of two papers:

1. Professional Dilemma Paper: this is similar to a situational judgement examination and requires individuals to think about how to act as a doctor in particular situations. More specifically, it requires candidates to demonstrate integrity, coping under pressure, sensitivity, empathy and recognising and prioritising their workload.

2. Clinical Problem-Solving Paper: this assesses 12 different subject areas (Cardiovascular, Dermatology/ENT/Ophthalmology, Endocrine/Metabolic, Gastroenterology/Nutrition, Infectious Diseases/Haematology/Immunology/Allergies/Genetics, Musculoskeletal, Paediatrics, Pharmacology, Psychiatry/Neurology, Renal/Urology, Reproductive/Obstetrics and Gynaecology, Respiratory).
Questions are focused on investigations, diagnosis, emergencies, prescribing and management.

The score from the MSRA exam makes up 60% of the overall score. The MSRA is a computer based exam and can be taken in the UK or abroad in a Pearson VUE centre. Those who score in the top 10% of the cohort will be given a direct specialty training job offer.

4. Selection centre interview

This is a face-to-face interview, in which candidates present a portfolio and explain why they have chosen a career in general practice. There are three simulated consultation stations with actors and one written prioritisation question. The focus is on communication skills in all aspects of the interview process. The interview makes up 40% of the overall score.

After this, the candidate is ranked according to their overall performance with scores in the MSRA exam and interview combined.

5. **Successful offer for GP specialty training**

The offer for a GP training post is made via ORIEL with a 48 hours timescale to respond to the offer with the options: ACCEPT, DECLINE or HOLD.

Entry requirements for the GP register

1. Completed a minimum of three years General Practitioner Specialty Training (GPST) on a GMC approved programme (usually 18 months in general practices, 18 months in hospital settings)
2. A PASS in the Membership of the Royal College of General Practitioners (MRCGP)
3. A Certificate of Completion of Training

Doctors who move to the UK from abroad are expected to demonstrate equivalent knowledge, experience and skills to qualify for entry onto the GP medical register.

4. GENERAL SURGERY

What is General Surgery?
General surgery is a varied specialty, which encompasses a broad range of surgical procedures, including:
- surgical conditions of the gastrointestinal tract from the oesophagus to the anus
- breast conditions
- kidney, transplant, and liver transplantation
- trauma to the abdomen and thorax
- certain skin conditions
- initial assessments of patients with peripheral vascular diseases
- general surgery of childhood
- elective surgery.

General surgery is one of the two largest surgical specialties in the UK, employing around 31% of the country's consultant surgeons.

What does a General Surgeon do?
General surgeons employ a wide range of knowledge and skills to perform surgery – as an elective or an emergency. Surgeons generally develop their own subspecialty, as well as performing more general work. Sub-specialities within general surgery include:
- breast surgery – assessment of breast systems, breast cancer surgery and breast reconstructive surgery
- lower gastrointestinal surgery – diseases of the colon, rectum and anal canal
- endocrine surgery – thyroid and endocrine glands
- upper gastrointestinal – oesophagus, stomach, liver and pancreas, incorporating weight loss surgery
- transplant surgery – renal (kidney), hepatic (liver) and pancreatic transplantation.

There is also the option to complete advanced trauma surgery and for remote and rural surgery.

Common procedures within general surgery also include laparoscopic or minimally invasive surgery such as 'keyhole surgery'. This technique offers patients a shorter recovery time, is less scary and can have improved outcomes. It has become a favourite sub-speciality within general surgery.

General surgeons work in a variety of areas, as well as playing an important part in emergency departments where emergency surgery is necessary. They are required to work as part of the multidisciplinary team, taking a holistic approach to treatment.

Entry Requirements for General Surgery Training

Dr Yazdan has extracted interesting information from the useful sources listed below, to guide you the reader as to the entry requirements and application process for this medical specialty.

See these **Useful sources:**

1. Supplementary Applicant Handbook, 2021 Core Surgical Training – Health Education England - https://coresurgeryinterview.com/resources/CST--Supplementary-Applicant-Handbook---2021.pdf

2. Self-Assessment Scoring Guidance for Candidates, 2021 Core Surgical Training – Health Education England - https://coresurgeryinterview.com/resources/2021-Self-Assessment-Guidance-for-Candidates..pdf

3. Royal College of Surgeons of England - https://www.rcseng.ac.uk

4. Person Specification General Surgery ST1 – Health Education England. https://specialtytraining.hee.nhs.uk/portals/1/Content/Person%20Specifications/Core%20Surgical%20Training/CORE%20SURGICAL%20TRAINING%20-%20CT1%202021.pdf

Essential
1. Applicants must hold an MBBS or equivalent medical qualification.
2. Applicants must be eligible for full registration with licence to practise from the GMC at the intended start date.
3. Completion of the UK Foundation Programme or 12 months experiences after full GMC registration or equivalent and evidence of achievement of Foundation competencies in the three years preceding the intended start date from a UK Foundation Programme or equivalent, in line with GMC standards.
Desirable
- Degree of manual dexterity, good hand-eye co-ordination, excellent vision etc
- Good organisational ability and effective decision-making skills
- Excellent communication skills
- Emotional resilience
- Physical stamina
- Research and audit skills: evidence of relevant academic and research achievements, e.g. degrees, prizes, awards, distinctions, publications, presentations, other achievements; evidence of involvement in an audit project, a quality improvement project, formal research project or other activity which focuses on patient safety and clinical improvement or demonstrates an interest in, and commitment to, the specialty beyond the mandatory curriculum.
- Teaching: evidence of interest in, and experience of, teaching; evidence of feedback for teaching.
- Management and leadership skills: evidence of involvement in management commensurate with experience; demonstrates an understanding of NHS management and resources; evidence of effective multi-disciplinary team working and leadership, supported by multi- source feedback or other workplace-based assessments; evidence of effective leadership in and outside medicine.
- IT skills: demonstrates information technology skills.

- Other: evidence of achievement outside medicine; evidence of altruistic behaviour, e.g. voluntary work; evidence of organisational skills – not necessarily in medicine, e.g. grant or bursary applications, organisation of a University club, sports section, etc.
- Evidence of participation in extracurricular activities / achievements relevant to surgery throughout career progression. For example, membership of relevant surgical bodies/societies, attendance at relevant courses/conferences, surgical elective, logbook and undergraduate/ postgraduate surgical projects etc.

The General Surgery Specialty Application Process

1. ORIEL (application)

All applications are made electronically via ORIEL recruitment portal website. You will be asked to provide factual information about you and your employment history. There is a two-week window to apply via ORIEL, in which after this time you will hear if you have been invited to attend the next phase of the application process.

2. Self-Assessment Scoring (application)

As part of the application process, doctors are expected to complete a self-assessment score. Doctors must provide suitable evidence of all achievement in order to be awarded points. There is no set number of years in which the achievements must be completed, but all achievements must have been gained after commencing your medical degree.

Option	Score
MRCS Part A Examination: (choose one)	
I have sat and passed the MRCS Part A Examination	3
I have sat and failed the MRCS Part A Examination OR I have already booked to sit the exam in the future	1
I have not sat and have not booked an MRCS Part A exam	0
Attendance at Surgical Courses: (choose one)	
I have attended two or more surgical courses	4
I have attended one surgical course	2
I have not attended any surgical courses	0
Surgical Experience: (choose one)	
Involvement in 15 cases or more	3

Involvement in 11-14 cases	2
Involvement in 5-10 cases	1
No evidence/involved in <5 cases	0
Completion of a surgical taster: (choose one)	
I have attended 4 to 5 days of surgical taster sessions	3
I have attended 1 to 3 days of surgical taster sessions	1
I have not attended/have attended <1 day of a surgical taster	0
Completion of a surgical elective: (choose one)	
I have undertaken an elective in a surgical specialty	3
I have not undertaken an elective in a surgical specialty	0
Post-graduate degree and qualifications and additional degrees:	
PhD or MD by additional research	4
Bachelor's degree in addition to primary medical qualification	4
Taught and research Master's degree	3
Single-year post-graduate course	2
MPhil	2
Degree obtained during medical course (2:1 or above)	2
Any other degrees or qualifications in addition to primary medical qualification	1
Primary medical qualification only	1
Prizes/Awards	
Awarded national prize related to medicine	8
High-achievement award for primary medical qualification	6
More than one prize / distinction/ merit related to parts of the medical course or Foundation Programme awarded to no more than the top 20%	4
Awarded regional prize related to medicine	4
One prize / distinction / merit related to parts of the medical course or foundation training awarded to no more than the top 20%	3
Awarded local prize related to medicine	2
Scholarship / bursary / equivalent awarded during medical undergraduate training or Foundation training	2
None/other	0
Quality Improvement (QI)/Clinical Audit	
I played a leading role in the design and implementation of a sustainable change (I.e., more than one completed cycle) using QI methodology or clinical audit and I have presented the complete results at a regional or national meeting.	11
I played a leading role in the design and implementation of a sustainable change (i.e. more than one completed cycle) using QI methodology or clinical audit and I have presented the complete results at a local meeting.	9
I played a leading role in the design and implementation of a sustainable change (i.e., more than one completed cycle) using QI methodology or clinical audit, but I have not presented the results.	8

I have actively participated in the design and implementation of a sustainable change (i.e., more than one completed cycle) using QI methodology or clinical audit, and I have presented the complete results at a meeting.	6
I have actively participated in the design and implementation of a sustainable (i.e., more than one completed cycle) change using QI methodology or clinical audit, but I have not presented the complete results at a meeting.	4
I have participated only in certain stages of a quality improvement project or clinical audit, which has completed at least one cycle.	2
None/other	0
Teaching Experience	
I have worked with local tutors to design and organise a teaching programme (a series of sessions) to enhance organised teaching for healthcare professionals or medical students at a regional level. AND I have contributed regularly to teaching over a period of approximately three months or longer. AND I have evidence of formal feedback.	8
I have worked with local tutors to design and organise a teaching programme (a series of sessions) to enhance organised teaching for healthcare professionals or medical students at a local level. AND I have contributed regularly to teaching over a period of approximately three months or longer. AND I have evidence of formal feedback.	6
I have provided regular teaching for healthcare professionals or medical students over a period of approximately three months or longer and I have evidence of formal feedback.	4
I have taught medical students or other healthcare professionals occasionally and I have evidence of formal feedback.	2
I have taught medical students or other healthcare professionals occasionally, but I have no formal feedback.	1
None/other	0
Presentations	
I have given an oral presentation at a national or international medical meeting after being invited/ selected to do so.	6
I have shown more than one poster at national or international medical meetings after being invited/ selected to do so.	5
I have shown one poster at a national or international medical meeting after being invited/ selected to do so.	4
I have given an oral presentation at a regional medical meeting after being invited/ selected to do so.	4
I have shown one or more posters at a regional medical meeting(s) after being invited/ selected to do so.	2
I have given an oral presentation, or shown one or more posters at a local medical meeting(s) after being invited/ selected to do so.	2

None/other	0
Publications	
I am first author, or joint-first author of two or more PubMed-cited original research publications (or in press).	7
I am co-author of two or more PubMed-cited original research publications (or in press).	6
I am first author, or joint-first author, of one PubMed-cited original research publication (or in press).	6
I have written at least 50% of a book related to medicine (this does not include self-published books).	6
I am co-author of one PubMed-cited original research publication (or in press).	4
I am first author, joint-first author, or co-author of more than one PubMed-cited other publication (or in press) such as editorials, reviews, case reports, letters, etc.	4
I have written a chapter of a book related to medicine in its broadest sense (this does not include self-published books).	4
I am first author, joint-first author, or co-author of one PubMed-cited other publication (or in press) such as an editorial, review, case report, letter, etc.	2
None/other	0
Leadership and Management	
I hold/have held a national leadership or managerial role related to the provision of healthcare for 6 or more months and can demonstrate a positive impact.	8
I hold/have held a national leadership or managerial role in a non-medical voluntary capacity for 6 or more months and can demonstrate a positive impact.	8
I hold/have held a regional leadership or managerial role related to the provision of healthcare for 6 or more months and can demonstrate a positive impact.	6
I hold/have held a regional leadership or managerial role in a non-medical voluntary capacity for 6 or more months and can demonstrate a positive impact.	6
I hold/have held a local leadership or managerial role related to the provision of healthcare for 6 or more months and can demonstrate a positive impact.	4
I hold/have held a local leadership or managerial role in a non-medical voluntary capacity for 6 or more months and can demonstrate a positive impact.	4
None/other	0

3. Interview

If a doctor's application is successful, they will be long listed and an interview will be offered. Applicants are required to individually book interviews on the ORIEL portal via a first come, first served basis. The interview consists of one 20-minutes interview station with two sections:
- management question lasting for 10 minutes
- clinical scenarios lasting for 10 minutes.

The panel consists of two consultants and panel members are the same for both sections.

Management Section
- one pre-prepared three-minutes presentation
- two minutes of questioning on presentation
- one management scenario question
- five minutes allowed to answer questions.

Clinical Section
- two clinical scenario questions lasting five minutes each. These are provided during the interview.

The interview is scored in these two sections. The management section is scored on content, presentation skills, questioning, probity and professional integrity, judgement under pressure and prioritisation and communication. Clinical scenarios are judged on clinical skills and knowledge, judgement under pressure and prioritisation, and communication.

4. Preferencing

Preferencing of post will be made available prior to offers being made. It is important you only rank areas which you will be willing to work in. For example, no. 1 is considered to be the preferred choice, no.2 is your next most wanted etc. If you do not wish to work in a particular area, you must indicate 'not wanted'.

Choosing preferences takes careful consideration, as general surgery specialty training is an eight-year programme and may determine where candidates practise in the future.

5. Offers

From this, applicants will receive a total score and a unique ranking will be determined unsuccessful or successful. Applicants will be informed via ORIEL. Offers will be made to those successful applicants that have 'matched' to a post and will be based on the applicants ranking and preferences. Applicants will then have the decision whether to accept, reject or hold their offer.

General Surgery Training

Core Surgical Training
Core surgical training consists of two years (CT1-2) providing training in several surgical settings. During the first two years, trainees must take the MRCS to gain membership of the Royal College of Surgeons. Core surgical training provides a generic surgical training with the opportunity for trainees to undertake more complex training in their choice of specialty.

There is the option, if eligible, to apply for run-through training, which means that doctors will not need to reapply for training at ST3 and will continue with general surgical training until ST8. Only a small number of specialties accommodate this.

ST3 Specialty General Surgical Training
ST3 takes six years to complete, progressing from ST3 to ST8. This is considered to be higher training, and evidence of completion of core training is necessary for entry.

At ST3 level the trainee will need at least 24 months' experience in surgery (not including Foundation modules). This includes at least 12 months on-call for emergency general surgery and can be gained in any country. Doctors may choose to work as a Locum Appointed for Training (LAT) or Locum Appointed for Service (LAS) after their core training, prior to applying for ST3.

Completion of courses such as:
- Advanced Trauma Life Support (ATLS)
- Basic Surgical Skills
- Critically Ill Surgical Patient (CrISP)

are essential for specialist general surgery training.

At the end of specialty training, trainees can apply for a consultant post after passing the Intercollegiate Specialty Examination (FRCS(SN)). A portfolio of experience which includes formal teaching, leadership, management, research, and audit must be completed too. Following this, a Certificate of Completion of Training (CCT) will be awarded giving entry onto the specialist register.

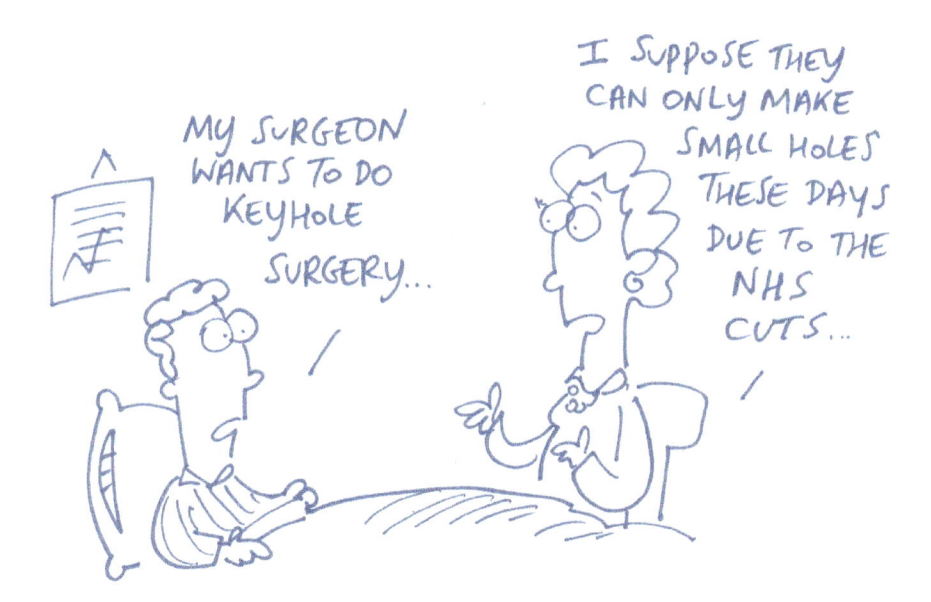

5. INTERNAL MEDICINE

What is Internal Medicine?
Internal Medicine focuses on dealing with the prevention, diagnosis and treatment of internal diseases. Physicians are trained to manage particularly complex or multisystem disease conditions that a single-organ specialist may not be trained to deal with.

In the UK, the four medical Royal Colleges are responsible for setting the curricula and training programmes:

1. The Royal College of Physicians of London
2. The Royal College of Physicians of Edinburgh
3. The Royal College of Physicians and Surgeons in Glasgow
4. The Royal College of Physicians, Northern Ireland

The Colleges are combined through the Joint Royal Colleges Postgraduate Training Board, and the process is monitored by the GMC.

Internal Medicine Training (IMT)

Internal Medicine training consists of a three-year programme, which replaced the two years Core Medical Training (CT1/CT2) in August 2019.

It involves gaining Membership of the Royal College of Physicians with a commitment to a chosen medical specialty.

Medical specialties include:

Group One Specialties:	Group Two Specialties
- Acute Internal Medicine - Cardiology - Clinical Pharmacology & Therapeutics - Endocrinology & Diabetes Mellitus - Gastroenterology - Genitourinary Medicine - Geriatric Medicine - Infectious Diseases - Neurology - Palliative Medicine - Renal Medicine - Respiratory Medicine - Rheumatology - Tropical Medicine	- Allergy - Audio vestibular Medicine - Aviation & Space Medicine - Clinical Genetics - Clinical Neurophysiology - Dermatology - Haematology - Immunology - Infectious Diseases - Medical Oncology - Medical Ophthalmology - Nuclear Medicine - Paediatric Cardiology - Pharmaceutical Medicine - Rehabilitation Medicine - Sport and Exercise Medicine - Tropical Medicine

Nature of the specialty

A career in internal medicine involves:
- diagnosing and treating a wide range of medical disorders that present acutely to hospital emergency departments and acute medical units, referring for specialist opinion and care as appropriate.
- providing advice and care for patients admitted to hospital under other specialties (e.g. surgery, obstetrics & gynaecology) who have, or develop, medical problems.
- diagnosing and treating the wide spectrum of medical conditions that are referred to medical outpatient clinics.
- managing inpatients and outpatients with co-morbidities, including elderly patients with frailty and dementia.

Common procedures and interventions include:
- advanced cardiopulmonary resuscitation
- direct current cardioversion (the procedure to convert an abnormal heart rhythm to a normal heart rhythm)
- temporary cardiac pacing
- insertion of venous lines (peripheral and central)
- aspiration of fluid from chest and abdomen
- insertion of drainage catheters into chest and abdomen
- lumbar puncture
- prescribing of drugs for acute and long term conditions.

Entry requirements for IMT

Dr Yazdan has extracted interesting information from the useful sources listed below, to guide you the reader as to the entry requirements and application process for this medical specialty. See these **Useful sources:**

1. Joint Royal Colleges of Physicians Training Board (about the specialty):
https://www.jrcptb.org.uk/internal-medicine#:~:text=Internal%20Medicine%20Training%20%28IMT%29%20forms%20the%20first%20stage,chronic%20medical%20problems%20in%20outpatient%20and%20inpatient%20settings.

2. Royal College of Physicians (applying to Internal Medicine): https://www.rcplondon.ac.uk/education-practice/advice/applying-internal-medicine

3. Health Education England Person Specification – IMT:
https://specialtytraining.hee.nhs.uk/portals/1/Content/Person%20Specifications/Internal%20Medicine%20Training/INTERNAL%20MEDICINE%20TRAINING%20-%20CT1%202021.pdf

Essential
1. Completion of a medical degree 2. Completion of the UK Foundation Programme 3. Portfolio/Application scoring 4. Virtual interview
Desirable
- Working effectively under pressure and making rapid assessments and urgent diagnoses - Managing and reducing risk including reporting and learning from errors, adverse events (including 'never events'), incidents and near misses - Stabilising patients, prioritising urgent clinical situations and referring patients appropriately - Using investigational resources appropriately (imaging, laboratory & physiological) - Communicating effectively with patients, relatives and other clinical staff - Advocating on behalf of patients where required - Leading and working in multidisciplinary teams

IMT application process

1. ORIEL

All applications are made electronically via the ORIEL recruitment portal website. The applicant will be asked to provide factual information about themselves and their employment history. There is a two-week window to apply via ORIEL, after which the applicant will hear if they have been successful in the next stage of the application. Applications are either short-listed, long-listed or rejected, against eligibility criteria; with the decision being communicated via email. All shortlisted candidates are invited to be interviewed.

2. Preferencing

Applicants for IMT specialty training, will be asked to rank regions in order of preferences. It is important to only rank areas in which you will be willing to work. For example, no. 1 is considered your preferred choice, no.2 your next most wanted etc. If you do not wish to work in a particular area, you must indicate 'not wanted'.

This requires careful consideration, as this is a seven-year training programme, and may determine where you practise in the future.

3. Application

There are two sections to the IMT application:

1. Eligibility section: this section evidences your right to work in a UK training programme, by completion of Foundation Training with details of your GMC registration. The candidate will need to list all rotations in which they have worked and provide contact details for three referees.

2. Evidence section: this section determines your score for the shortlisting process. Candidates must meet the following sections to obtain a good score:
   1. Undergraduate – whether candidates have obtained another undergraduate degree as well as their medical degree (10 points)
   2. Postgraduate – whether candidates have obtained a postgraduate degree (10 points)
   3. Prizes/Awards – relates to prizes/awards gained in medical school or thereafter (10 points)
   4. Presentations and Posters at conferences and other events (6 points)
   5. Publications (8 points)
   6. Teaching (10 points)
   7. Quality Improvement – completion of an audit, following the PDSA methodology, completing at least two cycles (10 points)

The application score is calculated from a maximum 64 points, derived from each of these domains, which contribute to the overall score.

4. Virtual interview

All candidates who are short-listed must be interviewed (usually via Microsoft Teams). The format of the interview consists of:
1. A clinical question
2. An ethical question
3. Suitability and commitment
4. Application and training

The interview score and the application score are combined to give an overall assessment score.

5. Offers

IMT job offers are made through ORIEL, and communicated via email.

6. OBSTETRICS AND GYNAECOLOGY

About the Obstetrics and Gynaecology Specialty
Obstetrics and Gynaecology are concerned with the care of the pregnant woman, the unborn child, and women's sexual and reproductive health. This combines both medicine and surgery and is a very varied specialty. Doctors working in obstetrics mainly deal with healthy women, but unexpected challenges happen frequently, such as complications arising in pregnancy. Gynaecology deals with the well-being and health of the female reproductive system, including endocrinology, female urology and pelvic malignancies. Special interests include high-risk obstetrics, fertility care or minimal access surgery.

Common procedures include:
Obstetrics: obstetricians undertake complex births, and intervene if the baby becomes distressed in labour. Their work includes:
- using instruments to assist delivery
- performing caesarean sections.

Gynaecology: procedures include:
- surgical interventions following miscarriage
- treating abnormal bleeding and polyps
- major surgery for gynaecological cancers
- surgery for endometriosis
- assisted reproduction.

Within the Obstetrics and Gynaecology specialty there is the opportunity to sub-specialise, including:
- maternal and fetal medicine
- gynaecology oncology
- urogynaecology
- reproductive medicine
- sexual and reproductive healthcare.

Entry requirements for Obstetrics and Gynaecology
Dr Yazdan has extracted interesting information from the useful sources listed below, to guide you the reader as to the entry requirements and application process for this medical specialty. See these **Useful sources:**
1. Health Education England Person Specification -

https://specialtytraining.hee.nhs.uk/Recruitment/Person-specifications

2. Royal College of Obstetricians and Gynaecologists (Applying for Specialty Training) - https://www.rcog.org.uk/en/careers-training/considering-a-career-in-og/applying-for-specialty-training-in-og/

Essential
1. Completion of medical degree 2. Completion of the UK Foundation Programme 3. A PASS in the Multi-Specialty Recruitment Assessment (MSRA) 4. Portfolio 5. Interview
Desirable
• Formal academic achievement e.g. intercalated degree, BSc, BA, MSc or PhD • Relevant experience in other specialties which would complement a career in Obstetrics and Gynaecology • Evidence of any relevant academic or research achievements, e.g. publications, presentations etc. • Interest in, or experience of, teaching • Management experience

The Obstetrics and Gynaecology application process

1. ORIEL application
All applications are made electronically via the ORIEL recruitment portal website. Applicants are asked to provide factual information about themselves and their employment history. There is a two-week window to apply via ORIEL, after which the applicant will hear if they have been invited to attend the MSRA exam or interview. This is communicated to them via email.

2. Preferencing
Applicants are asked to rank regions in order of preferences – including the ranking of areas in which they will be willing to work. For example, no. 1 is considered their preferred choice, no.2 next most wanted etc. If they do not wish to work in a particular area, they must indicate 'not wanted'. Choosing preferences takes careful consideration, as Obstetrics and Gynaecology specialty training is a seven-year programme and may determine where they practise in the future.

3. Multi-specialty recruitment assessment (MSRA)
The MSRA is a computer-based examination and can be taken in the UK or abroad in a Pearson VUE centre. This exam consists of two papers:
1. Professional Dilemma Paper: this is similar to a situational judgement examination and requires individuals to think about how they would act as a doctor in particular situations. More specifically, it requires candidates to demonstrate integrity, coping under pressure, sensitivity, empathy and recognising and prioritising their workload.

2. Clinical Problem-Solving Paper: this assesses 12 different subject areas (Cardiovascular, Dermatology/ENT/Ophthalmology, Endocrine/Metabolic, Gastroenterology/Nutrition, Infectious Diseases/Haematology/Immunology/Allergies/Genetics, Musculoskeletal, Paediatrics, Pharmacology, Psychiatry/Neurology, Renal/Urology, Reproductive/Obstetrics and Gynaecology, Respiratory).
Questions are focused on investigations, diagnosis, emergencies, prescribing or management.

4. Ranking
All candidates are ranked according to their score from their MSRA results, and then invited to be interviewed.

5. Interviews
The interview does not rely on a portfolio and consists of three stations which include:
- Clinical station – demonstration of clinical knowledge
- Communication station
- Structured interview station – presentation of achievements, research, continuing professional development, teaching etc.

The structured interview station matches up with the person specification for the role, which is available on the Health Education England website (see Useful sources above).

Essential	Desirable
Clinical skills	
<ul><li>Ability to apply sound clinical knowledge and judgement to problems</li><li>Ability to prioritise clinical need</li><li>Ability to maximise safety and minimise risk</li><li>Recognition and management of an acutely ill patient</li></ul>	<ul><li>Demonstrates aptitude for practical skills</li><li>Relevant experience in other specialty related to obstetrics and gynaecology</li></ul>
Academic skills	
<ul><li>Demonstrates an understanding of research</li><li>Demonstrates knowledge of audit, clinical risk management, patient safety, evidence-based practice etc.</li><li>Experience of active involvement in clinical quality improvement measures</li></ul>	<ul><li>Research and audit skills</li><li>Teaching</li></ul>

Personal skills	
<ul><li>Communication skills</li><li>Problem solving and decision making</li><li>Empathy and sensitivity</li><li>Managing others and team involvement</li><li>Organisation and planning</li><li>Vigilance and situational awareness</li><li>Coping with pressure</li><li>Values</li></ul>	<ul><li>Management and leadership skills</li><li>IT skills</li></ul>
Professional integrity	
<ul><li>Demonstrates probity</li><li>Capacity to take responsibility for own actions</li></ul>	
Commitment to specialty	
<ul><li>Show drive and enthusiasm</li><li>Demonstrate interest and knowledge of a career in obstetrics and gynaecology</li><li>Continuous personal and professional development</li><li>Evidence of attendance at organised teaching and training programmes</li><li>Evidence of self-reflective practice</li></ul>	<ul><li>Extracurricular activities in relation to the specialty</li></ul>

6. Offers

Following the interview, successful candidates will be made an offer to enter Obstetrics and Gynaecology Specialty Training.

7. PAEDIATRICS

What is a paediatrician?
Paediatricians manage medical conditions affecting infants, children and young people. The paediatric team provides care to patients ranging from birth to the age of 16 years old.

Levels of paediatric training and sub-specialties
Paediatrics is a highly sought-after for specialty training in the UK. The run-through training starts from ST1 up until ST8, with application and associated recruitment at ST1/2, ST3 and ST4 levels. The paediatric training pathway in the UK consists of three levels:
- Levels 1 and 2 are completed by all trainees
- Level 3: trainees decide whether to continue in general paediatrics or apply to complete their training in a chosen sub-specialty.

Level 1 (ST1-3) (2-3 years): paediatric trainees undertake Level 1 to gain a basic knowledge of paediatrics and child health, with placements in acute general, neonatal, and community paediatric posts. Doctors need to pass the Membership of the Royal College of Paediatrics and Child Health (MRCPCH) examination to progress into Level 2 training.

Level 2 (ST4-5) (1-2 years): training is usually provided in district general hospitals using existing core training posts and rotations that include community paediatrics and neonatology. Doctors at this level build their experience and expertise in relation to common paediatric conditions, child development and safeguarding.

Level 3 (ST6-8) (2-3 years): trainee doctors have the option to enter subspecialty training or stay in general training at this level of training. There are 17 different sub-specialties, other than general paediatrics, including:
1. Child mental health
2. Community child health
3. Neonatal medicine
4. Paediatric allergy, immunology and infectious diseases
5. Paediatric clinical pharmacology

6. Paediatric diabetes and endocrinology
7. Paediatric emergency medicine
8. Paediatric gastroenterology, hepatology and nutrition
9. Paediatric inherited metabolic medicine
10. Paediatric intensive care medicine
11. Paediatric nephrology
12. Paediatric neurodisability
13. Paediatric neurology
14. Paediatric oncology
15. Paediatric palliative medicine
16. Paediatric respiratory medicine
17. Paediatric rheumatology.

Paediatric cardiology is considered to be a specialty in its own right but is regarded as a joint specialty and so is overseen by the Joint Royal College of Physicians Training Board, with all other sub-specialties maintained by the Royal College of Paediatrics and Child Health.

Entry requirements for paediatric specialty training
Dr Yazdan has extracted interesting information from the useful sources listed below, to guide you the reader as to the entry requirements and application process for this medical specialty.
See these **Useful sources:**
1. HEE Applicant Guidance – Paediatrics ST1 -
https://www.rcpch.ac.uk/sites/default/files/2020-11/paeds_level_1_applicant_guidance_august_2021.pdf

2. Royal College of Paediatrics and Child Health – Specialty training at Level 1 -
https://www.rcpch.ac.uk/resources/specialty-training-level-1-application-guidance#national-recruitment-processes-for-2021

Essential	
	1. Completion of a medical degree
2. Completion of the UK Foundation Programme
3. A PASS in the MSRA exam
4. Portfolio
5. Interview
Desirable	
	- Ability to listen and communicate effectively
- Strong interest in working with people
- Ability to work in a multi-disciplinary team
- Willingness and ability to handle uncertainty and conflicting demands
- Ability to stay calm while working under pressure
- Excellent organisational and time-management skills
- Good IT skills
- Ability to manage change

Paediatric application process

1.ORIEL Paediatric application
All applications are made electronically via the ORIEL recruitment portal website. Applicants are asked to provide information about themselves and their employment history. There is a two-week window to apply via ORIEL, after which the applicant will hear if they have been invited to attend the MRSA exam or interview. This is communicated via email.

2.Preferencing
Once applying for paediatric specialty training, you will be asked to rank regions in order of preferences. It is important you only rank areas where you will be willing to work in. For example, no. 1 is considered the preferred choice, no.2 is the next most wanted etc. If you do not wish to work in a particular area, you must indicate 'not wanted', as paediatric specialty training is a 7-8- year programme and may determine where you practise in the future.

3. Multi-specialty recruitment assessment (MSRA)

This exam consists of two papers: the Professional Dilemma Paper and Clinical Problem-Solving Paper. The MSRA is a computer-based examination and can be taken in the UK or abroad in a Pearson VUE centre. The score from the MSRA exam makes up 40% of the overall score.

1. Professional Dilemma Paper: this is similar to a situational judgement examination which requires individuals to think about how to act as a doctor in particular situations. More specifically, it requires candidates to demonstrate integrity, coping under pressure, sensitivity, empathy and recognising and prioritising their workload.

2. Clinical Problem-Solving Paper: this assesses 12 different subject areas (Cardiovascular, Dermatology/ENT/Ophthalmology, Endocrine/Metabolic, Gastroenterology/Nutrition, Infectious Diseases/Haematology/Immunology/Allergies/Genetics, Musculoskeletal, Paediatrics, Pharmacology, Psychiatry/Neurology, Renal/Urology, Reproductive/Obstetrics and Gynaecology, Respiratory).
Questions are focused on investigations, diagnosis, emergencies, prescribing or management.

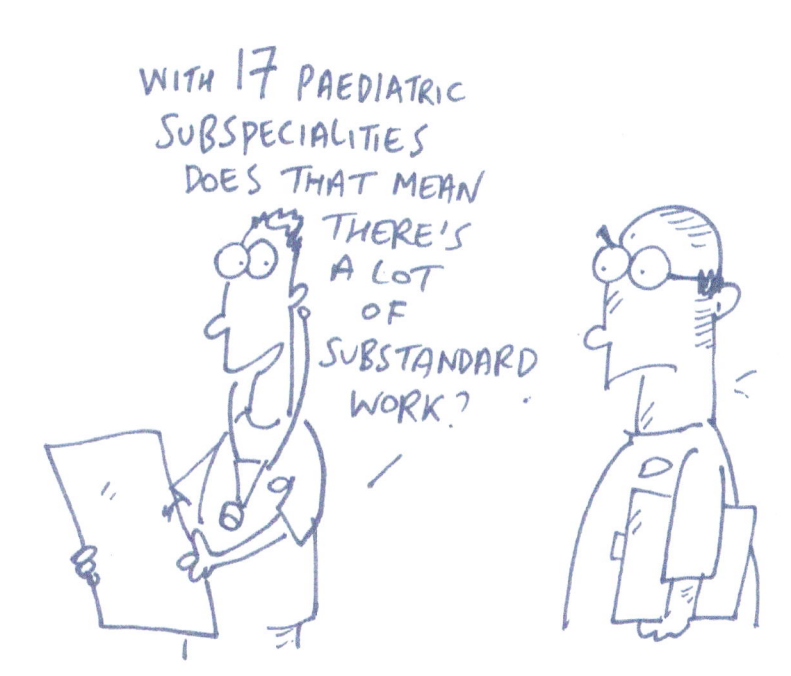

4. Online interview

All interviews are performed online on Microsoft Teams and are around 25 minutes in length. Interviews are assessed by two clinicians scoring each interviewee independently, against the following domains which capture applicants' clinical experiences to date and their understanding of issues relevant to working in the NHS:

- Communication (40 marks): the first part of the interview is used to assess the ability of the applicant to interact with patients/parents/carers. Applicants are given a scenario to read two minutes before starting their virtual interview. The scenario involves an explanation of a clinical condition or reasons for an intervention or transfer with interaction between the applicant and role player. The two assessors use a list of key points for scoring the content and overall performance of the applicant. Each assessor will score the applicant's performance out of 20, using a scoring framework tailored towards the specific scenario being undertaken, with positive and negative indicators to guide their marking.
- Career motivation (40 marks): applicants will *not* be required to demonstrate their portfolio but still prepare the content that they want to speak about during this part of the interview, which will help to demonstrate their enthusiasm, suitability, motivation and commitment to a career in paediatrics; as well as their understanding of the specialty and how their personal attributes and career so far will help to make them a good paediatrician. Assessors will not have access to any application forms during the interview (which will have already been marked). Applicants need to emphasise their career development and achievements in this part of the interview. Each of the two assessors will score the applicant out of 20, using a scoring framework tailored towards the specific scenario being undertaken, with positive and negative indicators to guide their marking.
- Reflective practice (20 marks): the final part of the interview will assess an applicant's understanding of reflection and how they apply that reflection to their experiences in medical practice for their career progression.

Applicants will be asked to reflect on a significant event from their career to date where something has either gone well or not gone well and reflect upon it to demonstrate how they will use their experiences to help them progress through their career. Each of the two assessors score the applicant out of 10, using a scoring framework tailored towards the specific scenario being undertaken, with positive and negative indicators to guide their marking.

Applicants are scored overall out of a total of 100 marks. To be deemed successful at interview, they must score at least 55%. After this, they will be ranked according to their overall performance in the MSRA exam and interview combined. Successful applicants will receive an offer for a paediatric training post via ORIEL, with only 48 hours to respond to the offer with options to ACCEPT, DECLINE or HOLD.

8. PALLIATIVE MEDICINE

What is palliative medicine?
Palliative medicine requires clinical leadership, care and support to prevent and relieve suffering for people with life-limiting and life-threatening illnesses. Its diagnostic and therapeutic purposes focus on meeting the individual patient's needs and preferences as far as possible, through shared-decision making and multi-disciplinary working. Expertise in palliative medicine includes:
- Assessing and managing physical, psychological and spiritual systems and managing distress
- Clinical analysis and skilled decision-making in complex scenarios
- Skilled communications and co-ordination of care
- Multidisciplinary working
- Care and support to those important to the patient, e.g. bereavement care.

Palliative medicine training
Entry to palliative medicine training is possible following successful completion of both a Foundation Training programme and a Core Training programme. There are five Core Training programmes for palliative medicine training:
- core medical training (CMT)
- acute care common stem (ACCS)
- anaesthetic training
- core surgical training
- general practice training.

Doctors can apply for palliative medicine specialty training after completing core training, at ST3 level, if they have passed the full Membership of Royal College of Physicians (MRCP) examination too. Following this, it takes four years training to gain a certificate of completion (CCT) in palliative medicine.

Palliative medicine curriculum
The purpose of the palliative medicine curriculum is to create doctors with both generic professional and specialty specific capabilities and skills, to manage patients with advanced, progressive, life-limiting

diseases. The focus of care is to optimise their quality of life, through complex symptom management and psychological, social and spiritual support. This is managed as a palliative care specialist and within a multi-disciplinary team.

The training programme for palliative medicine is competency based and is a minimum of four years in length. The curriculum covers a number of training rotations, where trainees receive experiences of palliative care in a wide range of settings, such as patients' own homes, day hospices, inpatient units and other inpatient specialist palliative care units, outpatients and general hospitals.

Further subspecialties/special interests can include oncology, chronic pain services and acute pain services, amongst others.

Entry requirements for palliative medicine
Dr Yazdan has extracted interesting information from the useful sources listed below, to guide you the reader as to the entry requirements and application process for this medical specialty. See these **Useful sources:**
1. NHS Physician ST3 recruitment - https://www.st3recruitment.org.uk/specialties/palliative-medicine

2. Association for Palliative Medicine - https://apmonline.org/

3. Palliative Medicine ST3 Person Specification -

https://specialtytraining.hee.nhs.uk/portals/1/Content/Person%20Specifications/Palliative%20Medicine/Palliative%20Medicine%20ST3%202021.pdf

Essential
1. Completion of a medical degree 2. Completion of the UK Foundation Programme 3. Completion of a Core Training Programme 4. Full MRCP (PASS) 5. Portfolio 6. Interview
Desirable
- Knowledge of, and experience in, managing a broad range of medical conditions - Understanding of, and appropriate attitudes to, ethical issues that arise in palliative care - Awareness of the importance of providing palliative care that is appropriate to the individual's cultural and racial background - Excellent oral and written communication skills in the context of liaison with other professional staff - Ability to work with individuals and families in crisis - Ability to supervise, mentor and support junior doctors - Ability to work independently but know when to ask for help - Ability to work and communicate effectively with a multi-disciplinary team - Ability to break bad news sensitively - Recognise own strengths and weaknesses - Recognises when stressed and has effective coping mechanisms - Demonstrate a high level of professional and personal integrity

Palliative medicine application process

1. **ORIEL**

All applications are made electronically via the ORIEL recruitment portal website. Applicants are asked to provide factual information about themselves and their employment history.

There is a two-week window to apply via ORIEL, after which the applicant will hear if they have been successful in the next stage of their application. Applications are either short-listed, long-listed or rejected, against eligibility criteria, which is communicated via email.

All shortlisted candidates will be invited to be interviewed.

2. Preferencing

Once applying for IMT specialty training, applicants are asked to rank regions in order of their preferences. They should only rank areas in which they will be willing to work. For example, no. 1 is considered as the preferred choice, no.2 as the next most wanted etc. and if the applicant does not wish to work in a particular area, they must indicate 'not wanted'.

Palliative Care Medicine is a four-year programme, and may determine where they practise in the future.

3. Application

There are two sections to the IMT application:

1. Eligibility section: this section evidences the applicant's right to work in a UK training programme, after completion of the Foundation Training programme, with details of their GMC registration. The candidate will need to list all rotations in which they have worked and provide contact information for three referees.

2. Evidence section: this section determines the individual's score for shortlisting. Candidates must meet the following sections to obtain a good score:
- undergraduate qualification – whether candidates have obtained another undergraduate degree as well as their medical degree (10 points)
- postgraduate qualification – whether candidates have obtained a postgraduate degree (10 points)
- prizes/awards – gained in medical school or thereafter (10 points)
- presentations and posters, at conferences or other events (6 points)
- publications (8 points)
- teaching (10 points)
- quality improvement – completion of an audit, following the PDSA methodology with the completion of at least two cycles (10 points)

For each of these domains, candidates are allocated points which contribute to their overall score.

4. Interview

The interview consists of six question areas which will last around five minutes. The interview will last for approximately 25 minutes. The four questions include:

- **Question One – Application and Training (scored as two separate sections):** application forms and training to date will be reviewed. Questions will be based on current achievements, and the individual's engagement with training and learning.
- **Question Two – Suitability and Commitment:** suitability for, and commitment to, ST3 training.
- **Question Three – Ethical Communication:** this station features assessment of an ethical scenario, and demonstrates the applicant's communication skills. It consists of a hypothetical situation, details of which are provided shortly before the question. The scenario requires the applicant to focus less on the clinical situation but consider the moral, ethical, legal issues, whilst demonstrating good communication skills.
- **Question Four – Professionalism and Governance (scored as two separate sections):** this question is a discussion of professionalism and governance, preceded with a short question for discussion of an ethical scenario to demonstrate their understanding of professionalism and governance in a given situation.

The interview assesses all six aspects independently, and for each aspect the candidate will receive two marks – one from each of the two interviewers – giving 12 marks in total.

Each of these marks can be scored 1-5; so with 12 marks awarded, the maximum score available in 60.

The interview is scored, using the following framework:

Mark	Rating	Assessment
1	Poor	Not considered appointable
2	Area for concern	performed below the level expected; possibly unappointable, subject to discussion and performance in other areas
3	Satisfactory	performed at the level expected during CT2; the candidate is suitable for an ST3 / Locum Appointment for Training(LAT) post
4	Good	above average ability; the candidate is suitable for an ST3 / LAT post
5	Excellent	highly performing trainee; the candidate is suitable for an ST3 / LAT post

The Raw Interview Score (RIS) is the sum of all the scores awarded during the interview, prior to any weighting being applied. If your application is assessed as appointable, you will progress to be considered for the various posts on offer.

5. **Offers**

Palliative medicine job offers are made through ORIEL, and are communicated via email.

9. PSYCHIATRY

What is psychiatry?
Psychiatry is the branch of medicine which is concerned with the mental health of a patient. It focuses on the diagnosis, treatment and prevention of mental health conditions. A doctor who works within psychiatry is called a psychiatrist, who has undergone psychiatry specialty training. Typical mental health conditions treated by a psychiatrist are:
- Anxiety
- Phobias
- Obsessive Compulsive Disorder (OCD)
- Post-Traumatic Stress Disorder (PTSD)
- Personality disorders
- Schizophrenia and paranoia
- Depression and bipolar disorders
- Dementia and Alzheimer's Disease
- Eating disorders, such as anorexia and bulimia
- Sleep disorders, such as insomnia
- Addictions, such as drug and alcohol abuse.

Psychiatrists may also provide psychological support for people with long-term, painful or terminal physical health conditions.

Stages of psychiatry training
Psychiatry training is managed by the Royal College of Physicians and psychiatry training consists of two stages in the UK:
1. Core psychiatry training
2. Advanced training in one (or dual) psychiatry specialties

Core psychiatry training
Core psychiatry consists of three years (CT1, CT2, CT3), where doctors undergo rotations that are four to six months long in various areas of psychiatry practice. Doctors are required to undergo outcome-based and learner-centred training, encompassing indented learning outcomes matched to a GMC approved curriculum.

During psychiatry training, doctors are required to undertake three years of Core Psychiatry training, which include:

- Child or Adolescent Psychiatry
- Forensic Psychiatry
- General Psychiatry
- Medicinal Psychotherapy
- Old Age Psychiatry
- Psychiatry of Intellectual Disability.

During these three years, the trainee must pass all parts of the MRCPsych examinations, as well as completing several workplace-based assessments to achieve their competencies.

Membership of the Royal College of Psychiatry (MRCPsych)

There are three papers included in the MRCPsych examination:
1. Paper A: An MCQ written paper. Trainees are eligible to take this examination once they are registered as a medical practitioner.
2. Paper B: An MCQ written paper. Trainees are recommended to take this examination after 12 months of experience in psychiatry.
3. Clinical Assessment of Skills and Competencies (CASC): Doctors are eligible to take the CASC if they have 24 months full-time or equivalent post-Foundation programme experience in psychiatry AND a pass in Papers A and B AND they have a sponsorship in place. That is, a post within a programme of approved training or successful completion of an Assessment portfolio, showing equivalent competencies to that included in their Annual Review of Competence Progression (ARCP).

Advanced psychiatry training

Following three years of core training, doctors proceed to advanced higher training, which is also three years long (ST4, ST5, ST6). Rotations are each 12-months in general psychiatry. If doctors wish to specialise further, there is the opportunity to sub-specialise or develop a special interest, including:
- Academic psychiatry
- Addictions
- Eating disorders
- Liaison psychiatry
- Neuropsychiatry
- Perinatal psychiatry

- Rehabilitation and social psychiatry.

There is also the opportunity to apply for dual training in advanced specialty training.

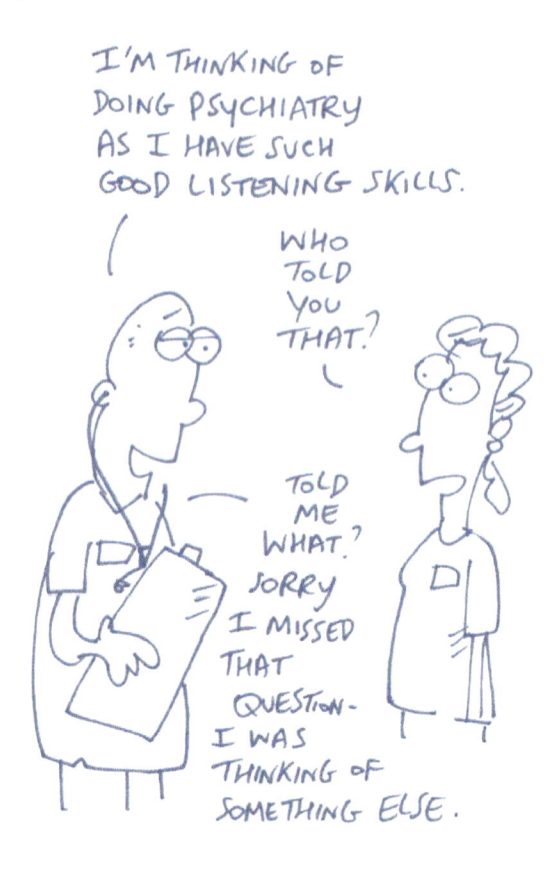

I'm thinking of doing psychiatry as I have such good listening skills.

Who told you that?

Told me what? Sorry I missed that question - I was thinking of something else.

Entry requirements for Psychiatry Specialty training
Dr Yazdan has extracted interesting information from the useful sources listed below, to guide you the reader as to the entry requirements and application process for this medical specialty. See these **Useful sources:**
1. Royal College of Psychiatrists – Your Training - https://www.rcpsych.ac.uk/training/your-training

2. Core Psychiatry Entry Requirements -

https://specialtytraining.hee.nhs.uk/portals/1/Content/Person%20Specifications/Core%20Psychiatry%20Training/CORE%20PSYCHIATRY%20TRAINING%20-%20CT1%202021.pdf

Essential
1. Completion of a medical degree 2. Completion of the UK Foundation Programme 3. Multi-Specialty Recruitment Assessment 4. Portfolio/application scoring 5. Interview
Desirable
• Make the care of your patient your first concern • Provide a good standard of practice and care • Take prompt action if you think that patient safety, dignity or comfort is being compromised • Protect and promote the health of patients and of the public • Treat patients as individuals and respect their dignity • Work in partnership with patients • Work with colleagues in ways that best serve patients' interests • Be honest and open and act with integrity • Never discriminate unfairly against patients or colleagues • Never abuse your patients' trust in you or the public's trust in the profession.

Psychiatry application process

1. **ORIEL**

All applications are made electronically via the ORIEL recruitment portal website. Applicants will be asked to provide factual information about themselves and their employment history. There is a two-week window to apply via ORIEL, after which the applicant will hear if they have been successful in the next stage of their application. Applications are either short listed, long listed or rejected, against eligibility criteria. This is communicated via email. All shortlisted candidates will be invited to be interviewed.

2. **Preferencing**

Once applying for psychiatry specialty training, the applicant will be asked to rank regions in order of preferences, only ranking areas where they will be willing to work. For example, no. 1 is considered to be the preferred choice, no.2 their next most wanted etc. If they do not wish to work in a particular area, they must indicate 'not wanted'.
Psychiatry specialty training is a 6-year programme and the area that they train in may determine where they practise in future.

3. **Multi-specialty recruitment assessment (MSRA) (computer based test)**

The specialty recruitment assessment is a computer-based assessment contributing to 33% of the overall total CT1 Core Psychiatry Training score (the remaining 67% comes from the interview). This assessment can be taken at Pearson Vue Computer Testing Centres, situated in a number of places in the UK. There are two parts to this section of the Specialty Recruitment Assessment, both aiming to assess some of the essential competencies in the national Person Specification.

Part one: Professional dilemmas (110 minutes)
This part focuses on a doctor's approach to practising medicine.
The candidate is presented with several scenarios and asked how they would deal with them. This test is designed to assess a doctor's understanding of appropriate behaviour in difficult situations, as well as allowing candidates to demonstrate skills such as professional integrity, coping with pressure, and empathy and sensitivity. Scoring is based on a candidate's responses and the appropriateness of their responses. The closer the answer is to that of the experts, the higher the candidate scores.

Part two: Clinical problem solving (75 minutes)
This part presents clinical scenarios, requiring doctors to exercise judgement and problem-solving to determine appropriate diagnoses and management of patients – and the extent to which the applicant applies

their knowledge and skills appropriately. Topics include those faced by a Foundation Year Two Doctor. Questions are presented in a variety of formats, with the candidate choosing the answers from a number of given responses.

4. **Interview**

All candidates who are short-listed will be interviewed to ensure that they meet the requirements of the person specification. Candidates are required to bring:
- documents to demonstrate that they meet the CT1 eligibility criteria AND
- a paper portfolio to evidence their achievements and show how they meet the person specification.

Interviews use a standard scoring framework with two elements:

1. Presentation of Portfolio Station (15 minutes)

A candidate's commitment to the specialty and learning are assessed in this station. Skills such as team-working and interpersonal skills should be demonstrated. Other assessment is based on academic and research skills, audit, teaching, organisational skills, communication skills and presentation skills. The applicant's portfolio will be presented to support this.

The purpose of this station is to allow candidates to demonstrate what has been achieved throughout their Foundation training, and how they meet the person specification for CT1 Core Psychiatry Training. Their portfolio should include:
- A copy of their CV, including previous posts and qualifications
- Their personal development plan
- Relevant workplace based assessments
- Any other supporting information, such as feedback from previous posts, patients, colleagues or references
- Reflective practice
- Audits / quality improvement
- Presentations / posters – shared at conferences or other events
- Publications
- Teaching delivered and teaching courses attended.

2.Communications in a Clinical Setting Station (15 minutes overall)
This station is split into two parts. The first section (ten minutes) focuses on interaction with a simulated patient based on a clinical scenario and the last section (five minutes) is a question-and-answer session, allowing the candidate to reflect on their performance in the clinical scenario.

5. **Offers**

Psychiatry job offers are made through ORIEL depending on the applicants' scores and are communicated via email.

10. PUBLIC HEALTH

What is Public Health?

Public health is concerned with helping people to stay healthy and protecting them from threats to their health. Public Health activities can involve helping individuals, as well as dealing with wider factors that impact the health of the wider population. The World Health Organisation (WHO) defines public health as 'The art and science of preventing disease, prolonging life and promoting health through the organized efforts of society.'

Public health, more specifically, contributes to the reduction of ill-health by improving people's health and well-being through:
- protecting people's health
- improving people's health
- ensuring that our health services are the most effective, efficient, and accessible to all
- academic public health which builds on the evidence upon which public health is based.

Public health combines the application of many different disciplines, including biology, anthropology, public policy, mathematics, engineering, education, psychology, computer science, sociology, medicine, business, and others. Public health is an essential element of integrated care systems (ICSs) which bring together the health service, the care services and the public health service to focus on prevention, cure, care and the health of the population, underpinned by primary care.

What is a Public Health Specialist?

Public Health specialists have a wide range of backgrounds, including some with a medical qualification, and others with an equivalent scientific qualification. Public health consultants are public health specialists with a consultant post: strategists, senior managers or senior scientists who provide the three main 'domains' of public health:
1. Health protection
2. Health improvement
3. Healthcare public health.

However, public health consultants may choose to specialise in one area in particular.

A public health specialist or consultant will be able to:
- deal with complex public health issues
- either lead or work with senior colleagues on the planning and delivery of policies and programmes which aim to influence the population at local, regional and national levels
- plan and lead evaluation programmes
- provide professional, evidence-based and ethical advice for the commissioning of health and care services
- lead on the gathering and interpreting of information
- work with a wide range of organisations.

Public health specialists are generally employed primarily by local authorities and Public Health England (PHE), but can also be situated within Universities, the NHS, Defence Medical Services and in voluntary organisations.

Entry requirements for Public Health Specialty Training
Dr Yazdan has extracted interesting information from the useful sources listed below, to guide you the reader as to the entry requirements and application process for this medical specialty. See these **Useful sources:**
1. Faculty of Public Health - https://www.fph.org.uk

2. Public Health Consultant and Specialist Roles – Heath Careers – https://www.healthccareers.nhs.uk/explore-roles/public-health/roles-public-health/public-health-consultants-and-specialists

3. Training and Development (Public Health Consultant and Specialist) – Heath Careers –
https://www.healthcareers.nhs.uk/explore-roles/public-health/roles-public-health/public-health-consultants-and-specialists/training-and-development-public-health-consultant-and

4. Health Education England Person Specification (Public Health ST1) -
https://specialtytraining.hee.nhs.uk/portals/1/Content/Person%20Specifications/Public%20Health/PUBLIC%20HEALTH%20-%20ST1%202021.pdf

Please note that there are opportunities for non-doctors to apply for public health specialist training too; so applicants for specialty training in public health come from a wide variety of backgrounds (e.g. nursing, research, teaching, environmental health.) Those without a medical degree, or those with a medical degree choosing to apply through the non-medical route must: have at least 60 months (whole-time equivalent [WTE]) relevant work experience at the time of their appointment, of which at least 24 months (WTE) must be in an area relevant to population health practice.

Essential
1. Applicants must hold an MBBS or equivalent medical qualification OR a first degree (1st or 2:1 or equivalent grade) OR a higher certificated degree (Master's or PhD)
2. Applicants must be eligible for full registration with a licence to practise from the GMC at the intended start date, have a minimum of two years postgraduate medical experience by the time of appointment with evidence of:
3. Either – current employment in a UK Foundation programme OR 12 months experience after full GMC registration or equivalent and evidence of achievement of Foundation competencies in the three years preceding the intended start date from a UK Foundation programme or equivalent, in line with GMC standards

4. Fitness to practise
5. Skills in written and spoken English
6. Health – meeting standards set by the GMC
7. Career progression – evidence of satisfactory career progression throughout the documented employment history.

Desirable
- Achievements/extracurricular activities relevant to public health

Public Health Specialty Application Process

The selection and application process consists of three stages – application, written assessment and selection centre.

1. ORIEL (application)

All applications are made electronically via ORIEL recruitment portal website. You will be asked to provide factual information about you and your employment history.

There is a two-week window to apply via ORIEL, in which after this time you will hear if you have been invited to attend the next phase of the application process.

Preferencing: once applying for Public Health specialty training, you will be asked to rank regions in order of preferences. It is important you only rank areas which you will be willing to work in. For example, no. 1 is considered your preferred choice, no.2 is your next most wanted etc. If you do not wish to work in a particular area, you must indicate 'not wanted'.

Choosing preferences takes careful consideration, as Public Health specialty training is a five-year programme and may determine where candidates practise in the future.

If an application is successful, the candidate is invited to a written assessment.

2. Written Assessment
Candidates are required to undertake numerical and verbal reasoning test, as well as a situational judgement test. The examinations cover:
Literacy – Watson-Glaser Critical Thinking
Numeracy – Rust Advanced Numerical Reasoning Appraisal (RANRA)
Situational Judgement Test
(all computer based, and multiple-choice questions).

If a candidate is successful at the written assessment stage, they are invited to the selection centre.

3. Selection Centre
This process involves a mix of scenarios, group work and panel questions. The candidate must demonstrate experience in public health, and the passion and enthusiasm to enter into the specialty. The Selection Centre Test elements include:
- Face to face interviews with each candidate interviewed in six short panels
- A written test of qualitative and quantitative analytic skills
- Group exercise.

Due to the impact of COVID-19 in 2020, the face to face approach of the selection centre has been replaced with a virtual interview.

Public Health Training
The main training route is to become a public health specialist, with those following the programme referred to as specialty registrars. Training takes five years, full time to complete. Trainees are required to gain experience in at least two different training locations, in addition to health protection experience, to ensure exposure to a wide range of organisational and public health issues. There is the opportunity to develop a special interest, including:
1. Health improvement
2. Health protection
3. Health and social service quality
4. Public health information and intelligence
5. Academic public health.

The curriculum itself covers nine broad competencies related to the three key domains of public health (health protection, health improvement and healthcare public health). There are three phases to the curriculum:
Phase One: Academic Phase – the first year of training is spent taking an academic course, as well as preparing for Part A of the examination.

Phase Two: After completion of Part A MFPH, trainees are required to undertake a three-month attachment with the Health Protection Agency. Successful completion of this results in being attached to the Public Health on-call rota; and time to start to prepare for Part B MFPH.

Phase Three: Allows trainees to develop special interests and attend special placements. These can include posts with:
- Local Authorities
- Department of Health
- Regional Health Authority
- Prison and offender health settings etc.

Assessment: MFPH; there are two parts to the specialty examination. Part A is intended to test a candidate's knowledge, understanding and basic application of the scientific bases of public health. This is usually completed in the first 12-18 months of the training programme.
Part B is a 'show how' assessment of the trainee's ability to apply relevant knowledge, and skills to the practice of public health.
This is usually completed with at least two full years of training left. The assessment responsibility sits with the local Health Education England office and achieved through regular Annual Reviews of Competence Progression.

On successful completion of the training, trainees are eligible for entry to the specialist register. There is also a requirement to become a member of the Faculty of Public Health in order to pursue a programme of continued professional development.

INTERNATIONAL MEDICAL GRADUATES (IMGs)

For a large number of overseas trained doctors and refugee doctors, information on the structure of the health service and the alternative options open to doctors may provide a vital first step to working in the UK. The organisation of the NHS will differ significantly from the health service that they are used to in their country of origin, or where they trained as a doctor. They need information about the principles underlying UK clinical guidelines and protocols, referral pathways, patient expectations, the career structure for doctors in different parts of the UK, the way in which doctors are paid, and initiatives such as appraisal and revalidation - as many of these doctors will find these elements confusing.

IMG doctors need information that is specific to their situation as international doctors. Such information should cover GMC registration as a doctor in the UK, work permits and the limitations that coming from abroad will have on the options open to them. Qualifications from different parts of the world should be discussed and the role of further training if needed. There are some reciprocal agreements in place with some countries.

This group of doctors will require information on how to do the Professional and Linguistic Assessments Board (PLAB) tests, a necessary precursor to working in the UK for many and, for those who first language is not English and their medical degree was not taught in English, the IELTS examination (International English Language Testing System).

International Medical Graduates (IMG) Routes
Clinically, there are three main options for IMGs in the UK:
1. To become a UK Consultant or GP
2. To work in the UK long-term without becoming a UK Consultant or GP
3. To obtain a short-term fellowship and then return home.

IMGs can take several other career paths e.g. academia, research.

1. To become a UK Consultant or GP

To become a UK Consultant, IMGs must be registered and on the GMC Specialist Register. There are three main routes to be accepted onto the GMC Specialist Register:
1. CCT (Certificate of Completion of Training)
2. CESR-CP (Certificate of Eligibility for Specialist Registration – Combined Programme)
3. CESR (Certificate of Eligibility for Specialist Registration)

To become a UK GP, IMGs must be registered on the GMC GP Register.*
There are two main routes to enter on the GMC GP Register:
1. CCT (Certificate of Completion of Training)
2. CEGPR (Certificate of Eligibility for GP Registration)
*It is important to note that IMGs without any postgraduate training are not considered to be qualified as GPs in the UK.

There are different routes depending on the training completed in a GMC approved training programme via the:
Specialist Register:
1. CCT (completed GMC approved training programme)
2. CESR-CP (completed part of GMC approved training programme)
3. CESR (did not complete GMC approved training programme).

GP Register:
1. CCT (completed GMC approved training programme)
2. CEGPR (did not complete GMC approved training programme).

CCT Route

The CCT Route is an approved training programme. If a doctor enters UK training in the first year (CT1 or ST1) and completes the entire training programme, then they are awarded a Certificate of Completion of Training (CCT). This route is suitable for those who have not undertaken any other postgraduate training and/or are new IMGs.

This pathway is not suitable for all IMGs. Doctors are suitable if they fit any of the following criteria:
- doctors who have not completed an internship and plan to complete an internship in the UK (e.g. Foundation Programme).

OR
- doctors who have not completed an internship or have not worked after an internship.

OR
- doctors who have completed an internship and have worked after their internship, but have not completed specialist training (residency) and are not overqualified for the target specialty.

OR
- doctors who have completed an internship and have started but not finished specialist training (residency), and are not overqualified for the target specialty.

OR
- doctors who have completed internship and specialist training (residency) but want to change specialty, and are not overqualified.

CESR-CP (Certificate of Eligibility for Specialist Registration Combined Programme) Route

Doctors can enter a UK training programme in the second year or later which is considered to be the CESR-CP; having completed part of a GMC approved programme.

This pathway is best for IMGs who have already completed postgraduate training in their target specialty. Doctors are suitable if they fit any of the following criteria:

- doctors have not completed internship and plan to complete internship in the UK (Foundation Programme).

OR
- doctors have completed internship and have not worked after internship.

OR
- doctors have completed internship and have worked after internship, but have not completed specialist training (residency) and are not overqualified for the target specialty.

OR
- doctors have completed internship and have started but not finished specialist training (residency), and are not overqualified for the target specialty.

OR
- doctors have completed internship and specialist training (residency) but want to change specialty, and are not overqualified.

The CESR or CEGPR Route
If doctors do not enter a UK training programme at all, they can still become a UK recognised specialist if they can provide proof that they have had experience equivalent to that of a UK trained specialist. To prove a doctor's equivalent training, individual doctors need to compile a portfolio of evidence to demonstrate achievement of all the required competences of the specialty. This is then submitted to the GMC for approval.

On approval of their competency portfolio, doctors will be awarded the Certificate of Eligibility for Specialist Registration to become a Consultant or the Certificate of Eligibility for GP Registration to become a GP.

The CESR route is best for those who have completed training and have been practising abroad for many years. Doctors are suitable if they fit any of the following criteria:
- doctors who do not wish to re-enter a training programme.

OR
- doctors who are unable to successfully get a place in a UK training programme.

2. Working in the UK long-term without becoming a UK Consultant or GP
Becoming a UK consultant or GP is not for everyone. Many doctors prefer to work in the UK long-term without this commitment or aim. However, there are a number of steps required for doctors to achieve and sustain this route:

1. Obtain GMC Full Registration. This is achieved by:
   - English language proficiency (IELTS/OET)
   - Pass in PLAB 1 & 2 or an accepted postgraduate qualification
   - Obtaining proof of internship, EPIC verification, and Certificate of Good Standing

- Apply for GMC full registration.

2. Obtain an NHS job. This is achieved by:
    - opening an account on the NHS Jobs website
    - submit a job application for ST1/CT1/JCF/SHO or SpR/Registrar/SCF/ST3* or specialty doctor post
    - interview
    - acceptance of a suitable offer
    - apply for a Tier 2 work visa
    - relocation to the UK.

3. Continuing Professional Development (CPD)
All doctors should maintain their continued professional development to practise as a doctor in the UK. This is achieved by:
    - updating and maintaining knowledge and skills through the CPD system.
    - undergoing annual appraisals and five-yearly revalidation.

3. To obtain a short-term Fellowship and return home
Many doctors wish to gain training experience in the UK to use to serve their patients back home and many IMGs consider this option. There are three main options for this route:
   1. The Medical Training Initiative (MTI)
   2. A GMC-approved sponsor (outside MTI scheme)
   3. NHS jobs advertised as Fellowships.

For IMGs applying for specialty training the process is slightly different from doctors who trained in the UK:

1. Obtain full GMC registration
Applicants must demonstrate their knowledge through successfully completing the Professional Linguistic Assessments Board (PLAB) examination; however, if applicants have any of the following qualifications, completion of the PLAB is not needed:
   - Primary FRCA examination
   - Certificate of the American Board of Anaesthesiology
   - Fellowship of the Australian and New Zealand College of Anaesthetists

- Fellowship in Anaesthesia or Anaesthesiology awarded since July 1999 (by Bangladesh College of Physicians and Surgeons)
- Fellowship of the Faculty or the College of Anaesthetists of the Royal College of Surgeons in Ireland
- European Diploma in Anaesthesiology and Intensive Care (EDAIC)
- Fellowship in Anaesthesiology awarded since 1998 (by College of Physicians and Surgeons Pakistan)
- Fellowship of the College of Anaesthetists of South Africa
- Doctor of Medicine or MD (Anaesthesiology) (by University of Colombo, Sri Lanka)
- Doctor of Medicine (Anaesthesia) awarded since September 2003 (by University of the West Indies).

2.CREST Form (Certificate of Readiness to Enter Specialty Training)

The following individuals can sign the competency form: consultants, GPs, clinical directors, medical superintendents, academic professors, locum consultants with CCT/CESR and confirm that this person has worked with you for a consecutive three months within the last 3.5 years from the start date of the post in question. Then apply for entry to the chosen specialty training programme(s).

Take a look at Box 3.1 which gives a specific example of entry to Anaesthetics specialty training for IMGs.

> **Box 3.1 Example for entry to specialty training for IMGs: Anaesthetics training**
>
> ***Passing the Primary FRCA examination***
> A pass in the Primary FRCA exam must be achieved to begin anaesthetics training in the UK.
> The exam has two parts (taken separately):
> 1. Multiple Choice Question Examination (MCQ)
> 2. Objective Structured Clinical Examination (OSCE) and Structured Oral Examination (SOE)
>
> ***Obtaining Anaesthetics CT2 Competencies***
> Proof of CT2 competencies must be demonstrated to ensure eligibility to apply for ST2 level training.
>
> ***Certificate of Eligibility for Specialist Registration (CESR) route***
> CESR is a route to be a specialist in the UK, without having to go through any training in the UK. The IMG doctor must prove to the GMC that the training they have received in another country is equivalent to that of the UK with the relevant supporting evidence. The GMC will then pass the application to the RCOA and if approved, they can be registered as an anaesthetic specialist.

References

1. Health Education England. Medical specialty recruitment update 2019-2021: posts, acceptance and fill rates
https://www.hee.nhs.uk/our-work/medical-recruitment/specialty-recruitment-round-1-acceptance-fill-rate

Chapter 4. Prepare for your specialty interview[1,2]

Completing the application form

For most posts, selection will be made by an appointments committee on the basis of an application form including a curriculum vitae (CV), references, a portfolio and then an interview with or without a presentation – as described in differing ways for various medical specialties in Chapter 3.

Generally at least two people from the appointments committee will shortlist the four or five (sometimes less, other times more) candidates for interview. They should have done the shortlisting independently of each other, each comparing your application letter and CV against the person specification linked to the job description. They will read your cover letter too, gauging your enthusiasm, and whether you have shown that you understand what the job is about. What are you trying to sell a future supervisor or employer about yourself? Describe these strengths in a succinct way.

Include a cover letter with your application if you can, that summarises how your experience, qualifications and interests match the most important job requirements of the post or training programme for which you are applying. Craft your cover letter to address the nature of the post or specialty training for which you are applying. Address your letter to a named person, if the name of the senior person connected with the appointment is given.

Your CV

Your CV is your shop window. It has to be good enough to help to get you shortlisted for that interview so that your undoubted qualities have an opportunity to shine through. Looks are all important, so make sure that your application has a well designed layout that will catch the eye of those doing the shortlisting, especially if you're expecting lots of competition for the post(s) that you are going for. Remember:
1. A poorly organised CV may be interpreted as evidence of you having poor communication skills. Think carefully about the layout. Ensure that your strengths are clearly presented. Do not be modest – brag!

2. Do not go into too much detail about your earlier years, but make sure that all dates are correct and there are no gaps to account for. If you have had a career break be prepared to describe and justify it.

3. Tailor your CV for each application. Identify important information in the advertisement and the person specification and catch the attention of those short-listing as to your suitability by summarising your key strengths on a front cover page. That's what the appointment committee really want to know.

4. Consider a competency based CV. Explain how it is that you are competent for the job that you have applied for. This does not concentrate on what posts you have held, but is more about what you have achieved. So it might describe for example, that you learnt basic surgical principles during your surgical house job, performed operations X, Y and Z unassisted in a casualty post, have been on a minor surgery course and are now on the approved list for minor surgery. Or for a more senior role, a doctor applying for a senior management post might describe the competencies they have gained in people and project management along a pathway in a series of hospital or general practice jobs.

5. Resist the temptation to say 'please see CV' rather than completing the application form in sufficient detail.

6. Spelling mistakes are inexcusable with word processed CVs. Get someone to proof read it for you to spot other errors. Otherwise these could be distracting for the reader and detract from the content of your application. Consider asking a senior colleague for their comments on whether you have organised your CV in a way that is expected for a particular specialty.

7. Keep your CV short and to the point- do not pad it out with unnecessary words or be repetitive. Use action words like 'Achieved' to start your sentences where you are describing your experience and responsibilities that you have held.

Preparing for the interview – for a specialty training post or other role

Once shortlisted you must be prepared to capitalise on your achievements. Increasingly candidates are asked to prepare a presentation on a given topic. This is your opportunity to give a slick demonstration of your communication, organisational and information technology skills.

Spend plenty of time preparing for the interview – and what you expect it to cover. Make sure you have all the details you need of the organisation to which you are applying and the specialty training programme or job you hope to take on.   Be able to describe your strengths and give illustrative examples. If you are asked about your weaknesses, think of one that might also be construed as a strength (e.g. humility) or a gap that could be easily rectified by your experience of working in the new post. Ask a supportive colleague or friend whom you trust to give you constructive feedback, to let you practise with a mock interview.

If your interview is virtual via video-call, make sure that you've got good lighting so that your face is visible and the panel/interviewer can see your facial expressions easily which are a crucial part of good communication. Look at the camera lens rather than the panel members when you're answering questions, so it looks like you're making eye contact. Dress as smartly as you would do for a face to face interview. Find a quiet room to do your virtual interview where you won't be disturbed, with good Wi-Fi connectivity. Using earphones and a microphone should help to make your responses clear and minimise any background noise.

For a face to face interview, make a great first impression when you enter the room for the interview. The rating of an applicant may be strongly swayed by their appearance, body language and voice in the first 60 seconds or so. The panel will be looking for someone who is:
- confident but not arrogant
- pleasant and can fit in within the workplace setting
- serious about the job
- energetic
- thoughtful

- punctual
- motivated
- good with their communications skills
- reliable
- honest and has integrity
- a team worker.

Some questions are predictable:
- Why do you want to work here?
- What experience do you have for this job?
- What aspects of your current job fit you for this post?
- What are your strengths – give examples – and ..... weaknesses?
- What skills do you bring to the team?
- Give an example from your previous career that shows you have initiative.

You will usually be given an opportunity to ask questions at the end of the interview – so use that opportunity to make a good impression if you can. Ask questions that show your interests – and see if you can gauge what opportunities there might be for further developments etc.

1. Speak to current doctors in training or the present incumbent if it is a hospital or primary care post and the key personnel in the department or practice. Consider meeting the clinical director of the specialty that you are hoping to join in a local Trust. Try to find out what the local issues are for the Trust or ICS.

2. Find out who is on the interview panel by ringing the administrative assistant or person whose contact details are given in the letter inviting you for interview, if that letter does not include the information. If you know who is on the panel and their posts, you can anticipate the type of questions they will pose at interview and prepare well.

3. Read a copy of the annual report of the Trust or look at the practice website, if you can, if your interview is for a particular post.

It will help you to gauge the size and strength of the organisation, as well as give you ammunition to ask intelligent questions.

4. Decide why you want to enter the specialty training programme or take the post, what you want from the post and what compromises you can make.

5. Plan some questions that show your interests. What are the research or teaching opportunities for example within the training programme or clinical post that you hope will be offered to you?
What opportunities are there for diversification to gain and practise other skills?

6. Do not assume the interview panel can remember the details in your CV - or have read it even. Emphasise your strengths and experience as you reply to their questions.

7. Prepare a short aide-memoire or handout that you can leave behind, so that they can remember which candidate you were. Nothing too ostentatious though. If you use PowerPoint in your presentation your handout should include a copy of your slides (in colour) for each panel member as well as a copy of any other achievement you want them to note.

The big day
By the time you are called for an interview, the panel will have already seen something in your application or selection process that makes them want to take a look at you. Remember this if you think you are starting to flounder and regain your positive mental attitude. The better prepared that you are the less likely it is that someone on the panel can bowl you a 'googly'.

Do not antagonise interview panel members by questioning or even arguing a point. But consider how you will fit into an organisation or medical specialty that does not think in a similar way to you. The interview may be the first time that you realise that you and your potential employers or the organisation or specialty are incompatible. Be honest with yourself and the interview panel.

Some of the points below should be relevant to your situation; not all will be applicable for all interviews. The interview is designed to test your reactions under stress to a certain extent. Often the interviewer is more interested in the way that you handle a question than the content of what you say.

1. Dress to impress. Old fashioned advice? You are trying to sell yourself as competent and capable. Having said that, be yourself and express your personality, you must feel comfortable.

2. The first few questions will be designed to put you at your ease and settle your nerves. Make eye contact, smile and look interested. If you can remember the names of anybody as they are introduced to you that is a bonus. Avoid saying: "It is all there in my application form".

3. Some questions are predictable. Have answers for:
    - "Why do you want to work here?"
    - "What are your strengths…
    - …and weaknesses?" If they ask this try to think of a weakness that you have adjusted for e.g. "I'm not very good at time management, but I am learning to delegate more."
    - "What skills will you bring to the team?"
    - "What is your vision for the way the post will develop….?"

4. Be up-to-date with current health and care issues. Read the medical journals and newspapers. Have a view.

5. Do not be put off by apparently biased questions. It is unlikely that the interviewer is really sexist or ageist or discriminating in other ways. You may have misunderstood. Sometimes humour helps.

6. Some questions can be unnerving if you do not know the answer. The best thing is to admit your ignorance but say how you would go about finding out: "That is an interesting question" "I would have to look that up/ask someone."

7. Find the balance between thinking before you speak and thinking out loud if you are unsure about an answer. Interviewers may be

interested in how you approach a question even if you do not know instantly what they are driving at. If you do put your foot in it, do not dig any deeper. It is okay to say "Actually now I think about it, that's a daft answer" and have another stab at it. Or ask them to rephrase the question for you (but only do that once in an interview).

8. Honesty and integrity show through. Do not try to second guess the 'correct' answer. Politics are unlikely to be overtly discussed but issues such as rationing of health care, private health care, how the ICSs will fare, maybe. Say what you think and try to justify it.

9. Some interviewers specialise in unusual questions which might put you off your guard. Have a think about how you might respond to:
    - What book are you reading at the moment?
    - Which famous people, past or present, would you like to invite to dinner?
    - Who was more important: Florence Nightingale or Marie Curie?
    - If you were stuck in a lift with the Health Minister, what would you say?

The presentation
(see Chapter 3 for guides for different specialty training programmes)
Think of a presentation as an opportunity not a threat, as a challenge rather than a problem. Try and see it from the interviewers' perspectives; it can be a very boring task to interview half a dozen people who may be very similarly qualified on paper. In a presentation you are in control and you can stress your strengths to the panel.

1. Your talk should be concise and well prepared. You should understand the task and stick to it.

2. Time yourself and keep to the time limit. It is surprising how long those short notes you wrote can last. (Conversely, you may find you deliver the talk much faster on the day.)

3. Try to make the presentation interesting with an appropriate use of visual aids. Only use technology that you are familiar with; it will be less likely that you make a mistake.

4. Practise presenting out loud at home. Ask a family member or colleague to hear you present and give you feedback.

5. Give yourself plenty of time to arrive and set up. Ask whoever is organising the interviews if you can give them a copy of your online presentation before the event so that they preload it for you.

Your golden opportunity
At the end of nearly every interview comes the question "Is there anything you would like to ask us?" This should not be met merely with a sigh of relief that the interview is nearly over, but grasped with both hands as your opportunity both to show your enthusiasm for the post and to find out some more details. Possible questions are:

1. You could ask about standards or developments: e.g. do they carry out regular audit, how are problem issues dealt with or what plans they have for development or extension of the service delivery?
2. How is the workload shared and what are the outside commitments of those in the department or team? For instance, are consultants on lots of committees leaving the incoming doctor to do a disproportionate share of routine work; do others in the team work flexibly?
3. Is there a team approach or is there a sense of autocratic leadership? This can be a tricky area to uncover the truth. A question such as "Who makes the final decision if there is disagreement?" may be revealing.
4. What is the availability of study leave? How are study leave and holidays organised? Is backfill generally available for staff on booked leave? Are there restrictions on how many can be away at once?
5. What is the information technology infrastructure and support like?
6. Does the department or practice have links with others for support or educational activities or other networking?

Referees

People usually think hard about whom they will nominate as referees. It makes sense to choose someone whom you think will speak or write well of you. However the influence a referee can have is often exaggerated.

The main reason for providing references is to ensure that there is independent confirmation of a candidate's work history and achievements. A reference generally indicates more about the referee than the applicant. References should be used to confirm what has been discovered through the shortlisting and interviewing processes. So usually a panel will not look at the references until after the interviews have been conducted; some organisations only obtain references for the preferred candidate after the interviews have been held. While the qualitative information within a reference may be able to make a difference if two candidates are very close, they are the least important part of the application process. A poor reference is not much help to the candidate, but a good reference is not much help to the panel.

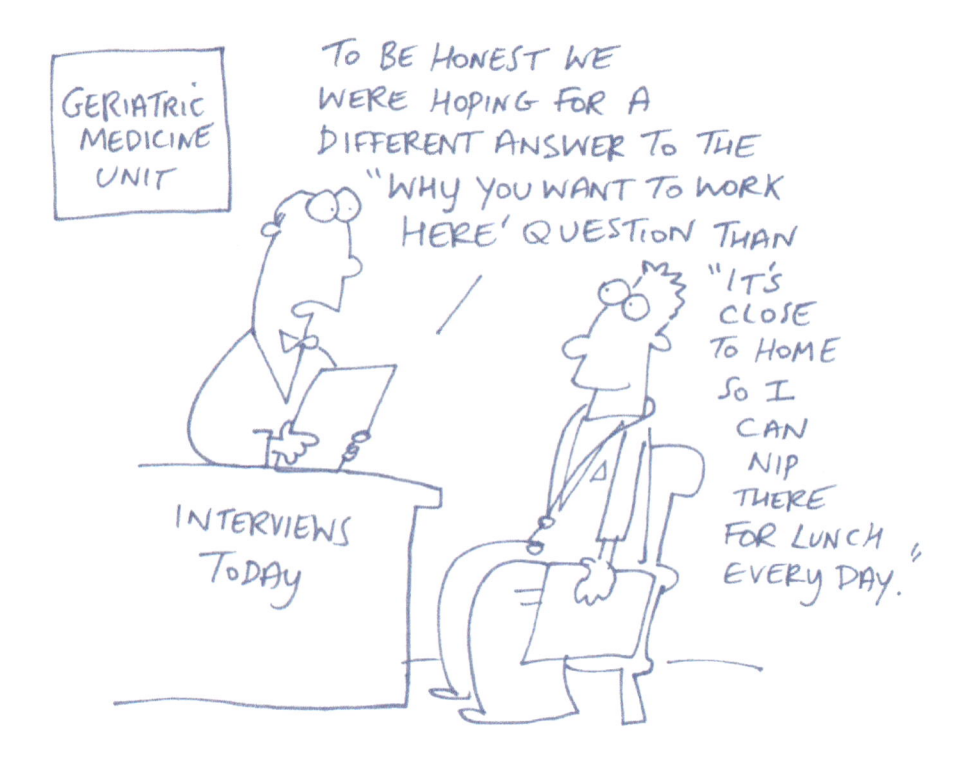

After the interview

If you are offered a place on a specialty training programme or the job you have applied for, you may be able to negotiate on some of the terms and conditions. If you are unsuccessful ask for feedback to find out why:

- Was it your CV?
- Was it how the interview went?
- Was it your lack of experience, skills or attitude?
- Was it because of the competition from other excellent applicants?
- Will there be other opportunities to apply for similar or related positions?

References

1. Chambers R, Mohanna K, Field S. *Opportunities and options in medical careers.* Oxford: Radcliffe Medical Press, 2000.
2. Chambers R (ed). *Career planning for everyone in the NHS – The Toolkit.* Oxford: Radcliffe Publishing, 2005.

Chapter 5. Making a career choice[1-3]

Job satisfaction and career fulfilment
Job satisfaction is known to protect people from the effects of stress from work. So increasing job satisfaction is one of the best ways you can recommend that someone 'stress proofs' themselves against the pressures and demands of a job. They will minimise the effects of the elements of the job they find more stressful if they enjoy their job, feel valued and are in control of their everyday work. Low job satisfaction can affect your performance at work too.

Career anchors: Consider what motivates you[4]
People are motivated by different things. Money, fame, power are all key motivators. Pride, lust, anger, gluttony, envy, sloth and covetousness are all listed as prime motivators - hopefully not all of these are relevant to any great extent for you working in the NHS! Some of the best motivators for fulfilling your needs are:
- interesting and / or useful work
- sense of achievement
- responsibility
- opportunities for career progression or professional development
- gaining new skills or competencies
- sense of belonging to a directorate or general practice team or the NHS in general.

Consider and balance the following features of work:
- balance between work and home
- job satisfaction
- working in a friendly atmosphere
- doing a worthwhile job
- prospects for promotion
- good financial rewards
- opportunities for flexible working.

Maslow's hierarchy[5] of a person's needs describes how self-esteem and fulfilment are not possible if the basic structure and safety components of their life are insecure. Fulfilment and personal growth are only likely to occur if the basics of a person's life are in place. Self-esteem, status and recognition from others are only possible if they are built upon a good social base that includes love, friendship, belonging to groups (work, home, leisure, professional), and social activities. Fulfilment, maturity and wisdom are only possible where all the other conditions encourage growth, personal development and accomplishment. If a doctor is contemplating a career change or extension of their career that will require new skills, knowledge and experiences, they might be better waiting until their personal life is reasonably settled and they feel secure if that's possible, before making major alterations or moving on.

Consider what is important to you as a doctor. The ability to critically appraise your own strengths and weaknesses, aptitudes and values as a person and as a healthcare professional is vital if you are to be successful in progressing in your medical career.

Integral to the process of career planning is having a real understanding of yourself: what motivates and what inspires you and what does not. Your life experiences, your principles and values, your relationships with family, friends and colleagues and professional identity influence your career choices. Therefore, the greater your self-awareness the more satisfying your career choices should be.

Your ethics set the boundaries as to how far you are prepared to go to get what you want. Work values are personal to you too. You will be happiest and most fulfilled in a job that incorporates your main work values.

Choosing the right career path for you

Everyone should take stock and review their options throughout their careers. Various triggers might occur in your life that prompt you to ask yourself whether you are happy at work, whether you are in the right job and whether it is worth rethinking your present career. Such as when:

- you are faced with a variety of opportunities and options, uncertain of which career path to take

- you feel that there is a mismatch between you and your particular career – maybe your personal ethics or values are threatened, or your needs and preferences have changed over time, for example if you now have children or expect to
- you feel demotivated or dissatisfied with your work – maybe your role has changed, or you feel that your career has plateaued for too long
- a serious life event occurs – bereavement, getting married, going through a divorce, developing an illness or disability
- a significant event occurs at work – a complaint from a patient, the traumatic death of a patient, you making a mistake, a critical incident arising from work such as you or a colleague being subject to a dispute or personal attack
- you are preparing for retirement – wanting to slow down for a while but not stop.

Life/work balance

Pursuing a fulfilling career should be about working smarter rather than working harder. The work/life balance is now as important to many people as any financial rewards. Working longer hours will not necessarily help you to work more effectively. Many people experience a tension between work and home demands and it can be difficult for them to juggle home and work priorities and set time aside to keep fit and relax. But you must try to achieve a good balance to give you an intellectual edge and help you to maintain your sense of perspective of your personal and work lives. It requires self-discipline to set personal boundaries, self-confidence to view your time as equally important to that of other people and energy to redesign your daily habits.

Career health is dependent on your physical and mental wellbeing and retaining a sense of proportion in terms of what is really important to you in life. Your career is just one element of your life, so do get it in perspective.

There are no hard and fast rules about how much time you should spend on work related activities compared to the rest of your life.

Sensible advice is to divide your day as:
- 45-55% on personal needs (including sleeping, chores, basic care)
- 25-30% on work
- 20-25% on leisure.

Only you and your partner at home know if you are getting the balance right. And if you have not got a 'partner at home' to discuss the balance with, maybe it's time you reduced your wholesale commitment to work and socialised more in order to make new friends. If you increase the proportion of work, it is the leisure component that is reduced proportionately.

Impact of your career on those at home
Do not forget the impact of your career choice upon your partner and family at home – if that is relevant to your own circumstances. Your family may not be tolerant of you prioritising your career, or studying for further qualifications or making a house move to take up a different post.

Factors to consider in *choosing* a career specialty or interest

When you review your current job or specialty, weigh up the potential for progressing along your career pathway or extending or swopping to a different role. Consider the match between you and the job as to whether:
- you have the sort of personality that fits with the requirements of the job
- you have the appropriate skills, training and experience
- you have sufficient job satisfaction and interest in your work
- you are sufficiently motivated to work effectively
- the job fits with your ethics, inner values and boundaries
- the job provides the balance you want between work and your off-duty life.

How will you know if you have achieved your career goals if you do not have a vision for the future?

Identify what you are aiming for and the nature of the milestones that will describe how you are going to get there.

This does not mean that you cannot change your career plan if your circumstances should change; it is essential to your success to be flexible.

Career crisis

A career crisis could be anything that abruptly alters the way you think about your career path. The factors that might temporarily or permanently derail your career can be divided into internal and external factors, and some are listed in Box 5.1. One example might be a doctor developing a physical or mental impairment that interferes with their work sufficiently for it to be difficult for them to continue in their post, or even put patient safety at risk. In that case they may have no choice but to stop work and revise their role and responsibilities within their specialty area or change career to another clinical or non-clinical position.

Box 5.1 Examples of factors which may affect the smooth flow of a doctor's career pathway

Internal	External
Illness e.g. short-term such as fractured limb; long-term such as depression or chronic health condition such as multiple sclerosis	Lack of career progression, lack of jobs
	Dealing with complaints that could potentially terminate career
Burnout	Immigration rules
Job dissatisfaction	Trust reconfiguration/enforced redundancy
Change of priorities, including positive changes	Discrimination (age, gender, race, disability, pregnancy)
Pregnancy	
Mismatch with intended career – personality, skills	'The establishment' – 'old boy network'
Self-questioning – "Is medicine for me?"	Family's competing needs – housing education, income, family illness
Sudden deterioration of chronic illness – not allowed to drive	Differing career paths of partner (geographic / time)

	Low income as e.g. part-time academic doctor
	Suspension and investigation by police after death of patient
	Being suddenly made redundant
	Complete change of work timetable by Trust
	Personal circumstances change e.g. divorce, bereavement

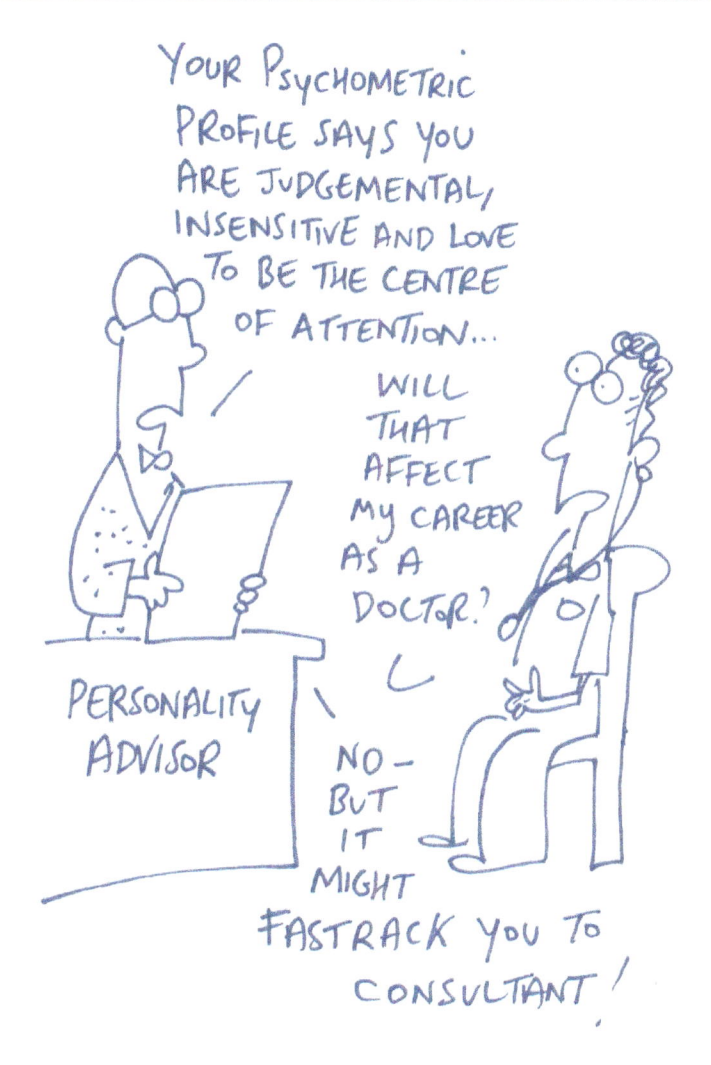

Your Psychometric Profile says you are judgemental, insensitive and love to be the centre of attention... Will that affect my career as a doctor?

PERSONALITY ADVISOR

No - but it might fastrack you to consultant!

Understanding the influence of your personality type[5,6]

Understanding more about their personality type can help people to make a rational choice about which career track they should follow. Career and personality match are very important – as are their personal preferences for their balance between work and leisure, work and income, degree of responsibility, type of work, and extent of interaction with people.

Knowing more about yourself, your personality and emotions, will help you to interact with and manage other people better. Feelings are highly influenced by your personality and your value system - all part of emotional intelligence.

Personality profile tests attempt to show individuals their preferred style of behaviour, in order that they can then choose the aspect of their profession that best matches the way they behave. Opinions about the benefits of psychometric testing are divided. The aim of the test is to identify a person's preferred way of behaving, based on their individual ways of perceiving the world and exercising judgement, in order to help in every aspect of life, career and personal relationships.

There is no right or wrong personality, just different personalities which work more or less effectively depending on the situation people are in. There is no ideal personality fit for a particular job and a mix of different personalities within the same specialty or workforce group bring fresh perspectives and balance to the work team. For many people, becoming more aware of their personal preferences and styles means that they gain confidence and pride in their own characteristics rather than seek to conform to an imagined stereotype.

Understanding yourself better will help you to realise your potential. The shy, inward looking person is not going to enjoy a work situation that calls for constant interaction, and the gregarious extrovert will become depressed if they are deprived of social contact. Understanding your own personal preferences and nature and what you want out of life should help you to embark on or develop an appropriate career path.

A poor fit between your personality type and the job you have might include you feeling:
- tired, stressed or depressed
- incompetent
- undervalued
- misunderstood
- unable to use your skills and strengths.

The common sources of stress described in Box 5.2 are those that people with different personality profiles (categorised by Myers Briggs[6]) are prone to. The more you understand personality-related reasons for any current dissatisfaction that you have with your medical post(s), the more likely you are to work on resolving current conflicts.

> **Box 5.2 Common sources of stress for different character types**
>
> Extrovert: too much time alone, solitary tasks
>
> Introvert: too many new people, not enough time alone
>
> Intuitive: too many details, lack of autonomy
>
> Sensor: uncertainty, lack of clarity, too much change, complexity, need to make long-term plans
>
> Thinker: emotional situations, disregard of logic, poor results from careful planning, hurting others' feelings while in pursuit of goals
>
> Feeler: conflict, giving too much, violation of core values, perception that a problem is their fault, hurting someone despite best intentions
>
> Judger: unexpected events disrupting careful plans, disorganisation, overwork
>
> Perceiver: tight deadlines or too much structure, situations where all options are closed.

Career anchors

Eight career anchor categories have been identified by Schein[4] to increase people's insights into their strengths and motivation as part of career development: these are technical or functional competence, general managerial competence, autonomy or independence, security or stability, entrepreneurial creativity, service or dedication to a cause, pure challenge, lifestyle. People define their self-image in terms of these traits and come to understand more about their talents, motives and values - and which of these they would not give up if forced to make a choice.

These help you to understand the meaning and implications of past career decisions and inform future ones, whether or not you work in the health service. They give you a clearer understanding of:
- your orientations towards work
- your motives
- your values
- your talents.

Career anchors will help you to:
- define the themes and patterns that are dominant in your life
- understand your own approach to work and career
- identify and clarify your talents
- provide reasons for career choices
- take action to secure a fulfilling career.

The questions listed in Box 5.3 will help you to identify your career anchors and prompt you to consider your areas of competence, values and motivation. Read through the detailed descriptions that follow and then come back to complete the Box. Fill in the middle column rating how important you perceive each career anchor to be for you. Then complete the right hand column gauging how you rate each career anchor in respect of the main job you currently hold. Add another column or two if you have a portfolio of other jobs and you want to think about each individually with a separate column for each.

Box 5.3 Identify your career anchors and how well you perceive these to match your current job

Schein career anchor[4]	How important is this aspect of your career to you (score out of 5 where 0 is *nil* and 5 is a *great deal*)	How does this feature in your current situation? (score out of 5 where 0 is *nil* and 5 is a *great deal*)
Technical or functional competence		
Managerial competence		
Autonomy or independence		
Security or stability		
Entrepreneurial or creative		
Service or dedication to a cause		
Pure challenge		
Lifestyle		

Is there a mismatch between what career anchors you rate as being most important for you and those that relate to your current role or career pathway?

Career anchor descriptions

Technical and functional competence: a high score in this area indicates that you value being able to apply your skills at work and to further develop those skills to an ever higher level.

General managerial competence: a high score in this area indicates that you value the opportunity to take responsibility for managing an element of the delivery of care or workforce support in relation to the organisation or medical specialty for which you work.

Autonomy and independence: a high score in this area suggests that you value being able to define your own clinical work in your own way. You want to remain in posts that allow you flexibility regarding how and when you work.

Security and stability: a high score in this area suggests that you value employment security or tenure in a job or organisation or future security. People anchored in this way are *always* concerned about how these issues affect them, and build their persona and career path to match these security and stability elements.

Entrepreneurial creativity: a high score in this area suggests that you value the opportunity to create an enterprise of your own (your own small business or project relating to your medical or other skills?), built on your own abilities and your willingness to take risks and overcome obstacles to reach your goals.

Service and dedication to a cause: a high score in this area suggests that you appreciate being able to pursue a medical career that achieves outcomes in keeping with your values and beliefs.

Pure challenge: a high score in this area suggests that you enjoy the opportunity to work on solutions to challenging problems, or find ways to overcome difficult obstacles in your clinical work or other aspects of your career.

Lifestyle: a high score in this area suggests that you value being able to balance and integrate your personal needs and interests, family needs with the requirements and demands of your career in your everyday life.

Being assertive

Assertiveness is about knowing and practising your rights - to change your mind, to make mistakes, to refuse demands, to express emotions, to be yourself without having to act for other people's benefit, and to make decisions or statements without having always to justify them.

It takes practice to be assertive - so get some practice in at work and at home. The biggest challenge may be being assertive with yourself so that you don't agree to take on additional tasks that are not essential for you to undertake, or that fall outside your own priority areas!

How often do you hear people saying: "No, no….no…..oh…alright then, I suppose so"? Listen carefully to what is being asked of you, weigh up the time, effort and skills the task or activity will take, and the extent to which it is an essential, desirable or possible feature of your working or home lives – and decide on your assertive response.

The chief points to remember about being assertive are:

1. Say 'NO' clearly and then move away or change the subject. Keep repeating 'NO' - don't be diverted.
2. Be honest and direct with everyone.
3. Don't apologise or justify yourself more than is reasonable.
4. Offer a workable compromise and negotiate an agreement that suits you and the other party.
5. Pause before answering a "YES" you'll regret. Delay your response and give yourself more time to think by asking for more information.
6. Be aware of your body language and keep it as assertive as possible. Match your tone to your words (do not smile if you are giving a serious message).
7. Use the 'broken record' technique - persistently repeat your message in a calm manner to someone who is trying to pressurise you. Don't be side-tracked.
8. Show that you are listening to the other person's point of view and giving them a fair hearing.
9. Practise expressing your opinion and rights rather than expecting other people to guess what you want.

10. Don't be too hard on yourself if you make a mistake - everyone is human.
11. Be confident enough to change your mind if that is appropriate.
12. It can be assertive to say nothing.

Support

Research into work stress has shown that people with the best social supports who interact well with other people, are able to cope with work or personal stress and are the least affected by it.

Be prepared to ask for help. That is not a sign of weakness or ignorance. Support networks may be used for another professional opinion or for emotional assistance. Don't be embarrassed or feel silly to be asking for help. A close and supportive spouse and family at home can be a good safe place to offload and share worries about work, so long as that does not stress your personal relationships unduly.

References

1. Chambers R, Mohanna K, Field S. *Opportunities and options in medical careers.* Oxford: Radcliffe Medical Press, 2000.
2. Chambers R (ed). *Career planning for everyone in the NHS - The Toolkit.* Oxford: Radcliffe Publishing, 2005.
3. Chambers R, Mohanna K, Thornett A, Field S. *Guiding doctors in managing their careers.* Oxford: Radcliffe Publishing, 2006.
4. Schein E. *Career anchors, discovering your real values.* Oxford: Pfeiffer, 1996.
5. Maslow AH. *Motivation and personality.* New York: Harper and Row, 1970.
6. Briggs-Myers I and Myers PB. *Gifts Differing.* California: Davies-Black Publishing, 1995.

Chapter 6. Career planning[1-2]

Your career plans may centre on developing your particular skills and interests within the specialty in which you are working so that you function more effectively. So:
- You may want to develop your career so that you become more specialised in a particular clinical or managerial area.
- You might want more variety in your work and decide to develop a parallel area of interest or a new skill that enhances your current post.
- It may be promotion that you are after with more status or responsibility.
- You may crave for a complete change; in a new career that is a natural extension of your current work, or as a fresh start in a different career within or outside the health service.

The medical educational environment is complex. Learning takes place in different places and at various times through a variety of methods and activities. The many settings in which learning takes place include lecture theatres, seminar rooms (online webinars, video-conferences), hospital wards, laboratories, libraries (in-person and online), consulting rooms and occasionally even in patients' homes. There are many factors that can influence the environment, including the socialising influences of fellow students, teachers, academics, colleagues, patients etc, and the sometimes competing aims of the individual, the health service, hospital or practice.

A recent national training survey that captured the experiences of over 63,000 doctors in training and trainers in the UK (that's 76% of all trainees and 32% of all trainers).[3] Despite the effects of the pandemic, 76% of trainees rated the quality of the teaching they'd received as 'good' or 'very good'; and even more (88%) described the clinical supervision they'd received as 'good' or 'very good'. There was some variation between medical specialties; for instance 95% of anaesthetic trainees rated their clinical supervision as 'good' or 'very good' compared to a smaller proportion in medicine (85%) and surgery (83%). Eight in ten trainees reported that they thought they were on track to meet their curriculum competencies/outcomes to successfully progress to their next year of specialty training or completion of training.

Many established doctors report that they have never received any careers guidance or counselling and any advice that they have received has been mainly informal and ad hoc. The inadequacy of the extent and scope of careers information, advice, guidance and counselling offered to medical students, doctors in training and throughout their careers has been widely publicised by academics and professional bodies over the last few decades; hopefully such support is more available now. Most rely on what they know about careers in medicine from personal experience.

Individual doctors should be enabled to manage their careers more proactively with dependable careers information available on up-to-date web sites, and improved access to impartial careers advice and guidance.

So for career planning doctors need to:
- be aware that they should continually develop themselves throughout their careers
- take responsibility for managing their own learning and career development
- develop skills to learn from all their experiences.

Career planning can be structured as in the three stages of Box 6.1:

Box 6.1 Checklist for a healthy career
- What do I *want* to do?
- What *can* I do?
- What am I *going* to do?

Careers information

You need *careers information* - for the facts about the qualifications and experience needed for alternative career pathways and the opportunities that there are for career progression. This includes written and/or verbal information about the number and type of posts available at various levels in particular specialties and fields, and details of the qualifications and training necessary.

The key to good career planning is information gathering from people, books, and general observation to capture the wide variety of jobs and opportunities available to doctors – getting ideas about what else to try and how to branch out - into a career in journalism, sports medicine etc.

Medical students and doctors need information about:
- the qualifications and opportunities for all sorts of posts or alternative specialties
- educational opportunities: bursaries, grants, new and established degree courses
- non-health careers.

Careers advice or guidance

Careers advice or guidance is personal and directive, providing advice within the context of the opportunities that are available. It is useful for those doctors who have not made a career decision or are unaware of the best way of achieving their career goals.

Such doctors might find it helpful to talk over where they are at with a careers adviser; this could be someone with a designated job in careers guidance, or it could be a mentor, a friend or colleague, an old tutor or local continuing professional development (CPD) lead. Someone providing careers advice or guidance should know about, and be able to provide, advice within the context of the opportunities that are available to the doctor.

Without adequate careers support they may remain ignorant of the options available, spend too much time in posts that are not ultimately relevant, and even be lost to the NHS altogether if they do not find the right niche and develop their career elsewhere.

The person giving advice or guidance should be well informed about the options and opportunities, and provide information or advice that is not biased. Trust managers may not give impartial advice to doctors about their career development if they wish to retain them in their current posts, or fill posts that fit with the Trust's or practice's priorities.

The quotes included in Box 6.2 reflect the lack of well structured and informed careers advice those doctors cited have received.

> **Box 6.2 Lack of careers advice and guidance cited by doctors**
>
> "Career advice usually happens after a chance conversation when you just start talking."
>
> "I need someone to invest in me as a person – someone who is interested in my existence."
>
> "Career advice is often perceived as something that anyone can do."
>
> "It's all word of mouth – it's who you know – everything is down to the individual."
>
> "One of the most daunting things of your Foundation Year 2 is suddenly having to put a CV together to apply for specialty training, completely on your own."
>
> "Medical school is one of those funny things. You can go there for five years and you have not really got a clue about thinking about jobs, how to apply, where to apply."
>
> "I have not thoroughly researched what each (specialty) involves, just what you hear from word of mouth around the hospital really."

Once established in a medical career doctors should:
- think carefully about taking time out from their medical career
- re-evaluate their career choice and why they are considering a change
- re-assess whether they work part-time or full-time or retire early
- match their strengths to a career specialty or way of working that suits them – e.g. taking on more responsibility, or extending their skills (e.g. becoming a practitioner with special interest or trying a secondment to management.

You need career counselling when:
- you are dissatisfied with your current job or career prospects
- you are unable to solve your career dilemma by yourself
- your thinking is clouded about your career and you need to talk things through with someone who is independent and non-judgemental
- you are not responding to the usual motivators at work
- you seem to be unaware of your talents and strengths at work.

Matching the components of a job with a person's preferences, strengths and qualifications, and their choice of career and personality are very important and dictate personal preferences for the balances between work and leisure, work and income, degree of responsibility, type of work and extent of interaction with people.

So reflect on the following sequence of challenges:
- "Who am I and where am I now?"
- "How satisfied am I with my career and my life?"
- "What changes would I like to make?"
- "How do I make them happen?"
- "What do I do if I don't get what I want?"

Any successful action plan needs a timescale and a description of what is possible in the short, medium and long-term. The outcome of career counselling should be *action.*
So a doctor aspiring to a mid-career move to a managerial role as part of their job portfolio for instance, needs to be aware of what areas their career development should span (see Box 6.3).

Box 6.3 Competencies for medical managers would include:
- Leadership
- Strategic vision
- Personal development skills
- Organisational management skills
- Change and project management skills
- Educational knowledge and skills
- Communicating, influencing, facilitating
- And many more……

A mentor might help you to develop your own thinking and find your own way, not teach you new skills or act as a patron to ease your career path by special favours. Being mentored should help you to realise your potential as your mentor should act as a trusted and experienced guide on personal, professional and educational matters; identify your strengths and weaknesses, explore options, act as a challenger, encourage reflection and provide motivation. Your relationship with your mentor should be one of mutual trust and respect in a supportive yet challenging relationship where the mentor remains non-judgemental. You might find that a supervising consultant or GP offers you informally that mentoring support.

A coach could offer you more directive help about your medical career in the same way that a sports coach urges an athlete on. Coaches can work through one to one conversations in person or by video-call or email or telephone. A good coach will be a successful motivator, be very supportive, establish a good rapport with you, be able to give constructive feedback and set clear objectives. A coach should stretch and challenge you and encourage you to solve problems and make changes. A good coach is analytical rather than critical and is able to depersonalise the problems discussed in coaching sessions by focusing on facts, outcomes and performance rather than personality or style.

You can ask around if your Trust or University provides any access to a coach or mentor, or if maybe someone knows someone who might provide you with such assistance.

Why doctors leave the profession
The main reasons that doctors leave the medical profession are that they feel that:
- they are not valued
- they are not supported
- they have an unacceptable work-life balance
- they are tired and overworked
- compassion fatigue (also known as secondary traumatic stress)
- burnout.

Many who do leave are interested in returning to practice if the circumstances and support are right with help and flexibility in designing their working patterns to achieve an improved work-life balance, with flexible or part-time working.

We need to remove obstacles faced by some doctors that inhibit their career progression. Many barriers are still prevalent within medicine today. These barriers to career progression play a part in some doctors' decisions to leave the profession altogether.

Doctors with disabilities or chronic illness face many difficulties. They are often stigmatised. They encounter inflexible working patterns, poor cover arrangements, little allowance in training or working for their health needs, ill-prepared colleagues who make the doctor feel guilty about the way their disability or illness impacts on their work.

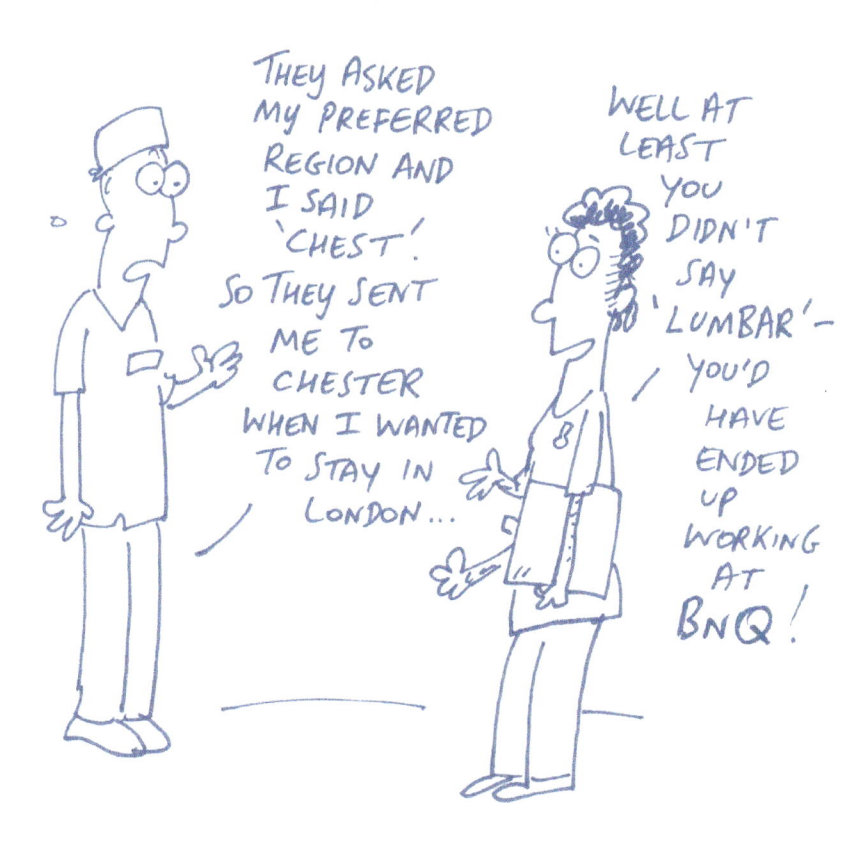

Doctors considering an academic career, may be deterred by financial disincentives (University employed clinical academic posts may have a comparatively lower salary than frontline clinical practice, but they bring an academic focus and personal growth without clinical pressures), the lack of a career structure and perceived clinical deskilling which is seen as a threat to resuming clinical responsibility.

Career planning is a lifetime continuum rather than an event which 'happens' in the early years of a doctor's career or when career difficulties or crises are faced. Doctors are keen to receive information and advice that is specific to their individual professional needs, and takes account of their family and personal situations.

Some training schemes and disciplines are more understanding than others about career breaks, and your careers information should give a broad indication of the differences in attitudes between specialties.

Careers advice and information sources

The NHS website that provides a range of information on medical careers is at www.nhscareers.nhs.uk/careers/doctors/. This site is divided into: working in the NHS, the NHS team - career options, and education and training. It provides information on career options, career path entry requirements, links to relevant organisations and case studies. The information is aimed principally at people considering a career in medicine, but does include some information for qualified doctors too. The British Medical Association and its associated journal have sites that give extensive information on doctors' careers in the UK. They include survey information and answers to frequently asked questions. Look at www.bmj.com, www.bmjcareers.com/, and www.bmjclassified.com/. They are an excellent place to start a search for careers information.

Online systems such as www.bmjcareers.com/advicezone offer an online enquiry service with previously posed questions and their answers available for all to read. Doctors can type in a search phrase and the system will bring up questions previously asked on the same issue. The answers given are specific to the original question, but doctors can extrapolate information for their own situation, to help in their decision-making.

JobScore (www.bmjcareers.com/jobscore) is a free online medical careers service created by doctors for doctors. It is an 'evidence based job hunting' system to help doctors make informed job choices from a peer reviewed database on hospital jobs throughout the UK. It provides peer reviews of medical jobs submitted by doctors who have recently worked in them. It covers all specialties, at all grades, in all hospitals throughout the UK. Those searching the site have to contribute at least one report of a post they have recently held.

References

1. Chambers R (ed). *Career planning for everyone in the NHS - The Toolkit.* Oxford: Radcliffe Publishing, 2005.
2. Chambers R, Mohanna K, Thornett A, Field S. *Guiding doctors in managing their careers.* Oxford: Radcliffe Publishing, 2006.
3. General Medical Council (GMC). National training survey 2021. London: GMC. July 2021.
https://www.gmc-uk.org/-/media/documents/national-training-survey-results-2021---summary-report_pdf-87050829.pdf

Chapter 7. Reflect on your progress as a qualified doctor and plan your career – yourself; using tools to understand and analyse the differences between career paths[1,2]

Try using one or more of the tools in this chapter. Our tips for any doctor managing their career are:
- Consider what you want or need from your career and what you can offer in return
- Recognise your transferable skills and the competencies you have already developed over time
- Develop one or more career goals
- Be flexible about change so that you can take advantage of opportunities as they crop up
- Promote an accurate profile of yourself – maximise your strengths, acknowledge your weaknesses or inexperience and what you are doing to address these
- Understand the value of your contribution to others and their work programmes in various health settings or organisations
- Plan for your future – never stop – even if it is to get ready for a fulfilling retirement.

A Stocktake on your Competence

Starting in the top left hand quadrant in the competency cycle in Figure 7.1 = *unconscious incompetence*. Here, you are blissfully unaware of your shortcomings until something happens to make you aware of them. That might be the realisation when you start working with patients as a junior doctor, that you are out of your depth now working in a medical specialty or ward on the frontline, and were not suitably prepared in your past training for what's expected of you now! It could be a recent patient complaint or adverse incident or it could be negative feedback from a line-manager, tutor or colleague.

Figure 7.1 Competency cycle

Unconscious incompetence	OBSERVATION ⇨	**Conscious incompetence**
Illness e.g. alcohol ⇧ out-of-date job changes too busy		⇩ LEARNING
Unconscious competence **(Expert)**	⇦ PRACTICE	**Conscious competence**

This realisation is a painful process, often referred to as cognitive dissonance, but until you become aware you cannot start the process of learning and filling those knowledge and skills gaps – as in the top right quadrant of *conscious incompetence* in Figure 7.1. Remember it's when you feel uncomfortable that you are just about to learn something and progress. Too much discomfort however can be demotivating and some people might give up at this stage if they feel there is too much to learn or they will never be good enough. Some feedback about their other strengths by a mentor or colleague would be a really good support at this stage.

The process of learning, with all that that entails, can then proceed and you will master the new understanding, knowledge, skill or task. You reach a stage where you know something new or know how to do something and can perform competently, so long as circumstances remain consistent - as represented by the bottom right quadrant of Figure 7.1 where you reach the *conscious competence* stage in your medical role. With practice and experience you then become expert. You can apply and modify your knowledge and skills in new situations that you may never have met before. At this stage at the bottom left quadrant in Figure 7.1, being *unconsciously competent*, you could teach others. It is also the stage when through familiarity, you can lose sight of your strengths, as your skills become automatic. Feedback on performance at this stage needs to include things you are good at so that you do not accept them as commonplace, you can reflect on them, keep them up to date and highlight them. In some ways feedback needs to take you from left to right across the bottom of the competency cycle to make you aware of your expertise again so that you can effectively teach others too.

It is possible to move back to unconscious incompetence from the position of expertise, in the direction of the bold arrow, through severe mental illness for example, or degenerative disease without insight, or even failure to keep up to date with best practice in your role or specialty.

Try Force Field Analysis

This tool will help you to identify and focus down on the positive and negative forces in relation to your work. You will gain an overview of the weighting of these factors. Draw a horizontal or vertical line in the middle of a sheet of paper. Label one side 'positive' and the other side 'negative'. Draw bars to represent individual positive drivers that motivate you in your role on one side of the line, and factors that are demotivating on the other negative side of the line. The thickness and length of the bars should represent the extent of the influence and perceived effects on you; that is, a short, narrow bar will indicate that the positive or negative factor has a minor influence and a long, wide bar imply that the factor is likely to have a major effect.

Take an overview of the resulting force-field diagram and consider if you are content with things as they are, or can think of ways to boost the positive side and minimise the negative factors. You can do this part of the exercise on your own, with a peer or in a small group in your workplace, or with a mentor or someone from outside your organisation. The exercise should help you to realise the extent to which a known influence in your life or in the workplace as a whole, is a positive or negative factor.

Make a personal or organisational action plan to create the situations and opportunities to boost the positive factors in your career and minimise the bars on the negative side.

Using a force field analysis approach helps people to identify and focus down on the positive and negative forces in their work and/or home lives and to gain an overview of the relative weighting of these factors. The exercise is suitable for anyone and everyone at any stage in their career to review their own circumstances and possible need for career development.

The next step is to make a personal or organisational action plan to create the situations and opportunities to boost the positive factors in your life and minimise arrows on the negative side – see the example in Figure 7.2. You could invite someone who knows you well to review the force-field analysis you have drawn and let you know honestly of any blind spots they think you're not aware of and have missed out and if you have self-rated the positive and negative influences on your working life in proportion.

Then it's time to decide which of the negative factors you will minimise and which positive factors you can build on, taking into account the needs and priorities of your home/working life and career plans – which can and should be addressed in planning for changes that you hope to make.

This can be done through:
- changing the strength of a driving force: width and length of the arrows
- changing the direction of a force: switching a force to be positive rather than restraining
- withdrawing or minimising a restraining force
- adding or enlarging helping, positive forces.

Figure 7.2 Example of force-field analysis diagram; satisfaction with current post as a doctor

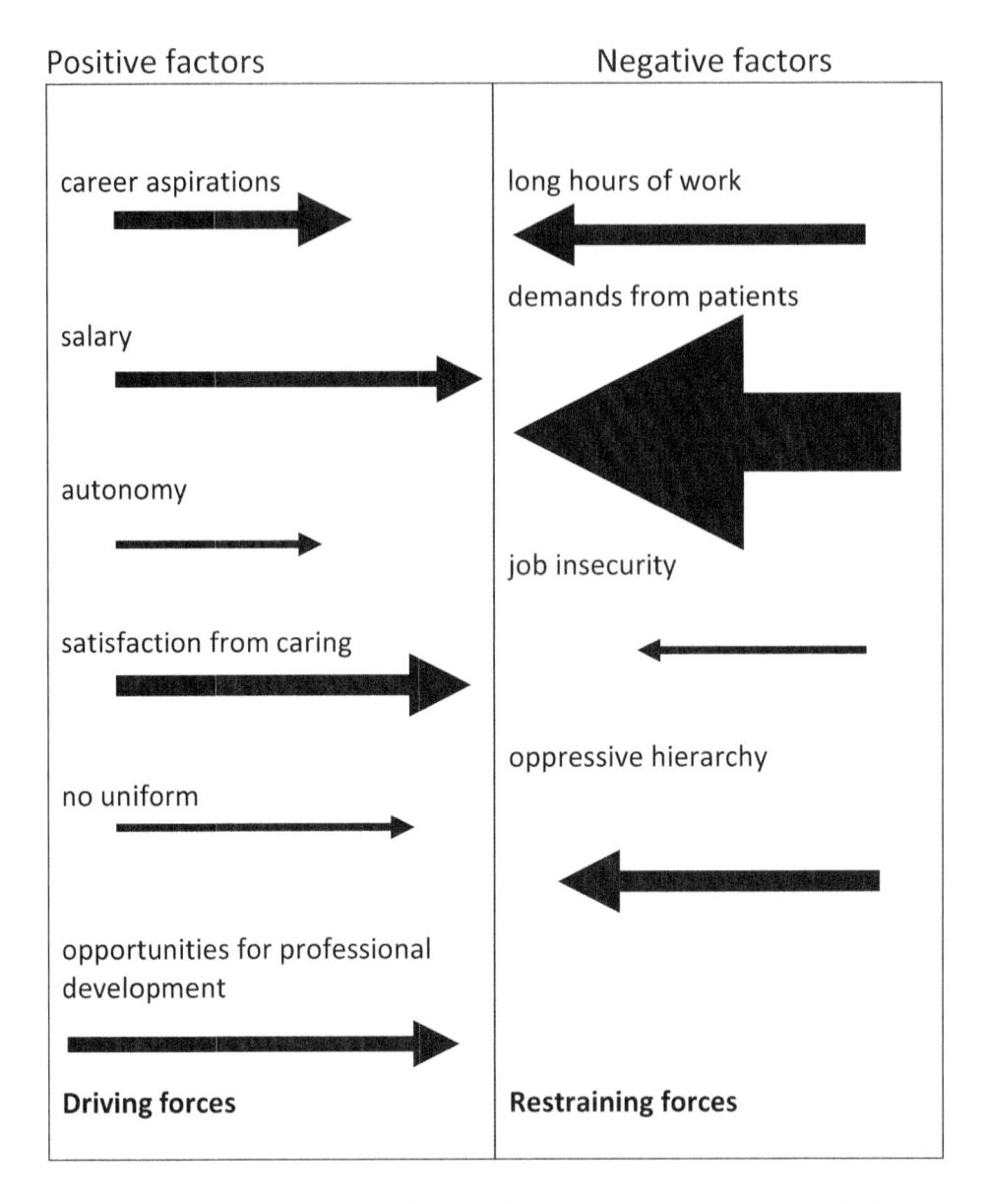

Positive factors	Negative factors
career aspirations →	← long hours of work
salary →	← demands from patients
autonomy →	
satisfaction from caring →	← job insecurity
no uniform →	← oppressive hierarchy
opportunities for professional development →	
Driving forces	**Restraining forces**

So now it's time to confront the gap between: 'Where I want to be' and 'Where I am now' – see Figure 7.3. This gap analysis is central to your planned programme of personal development and change; the nature of which depends on the various gaps identified and your future goals:

Figure 7.3: Outline gap analysis

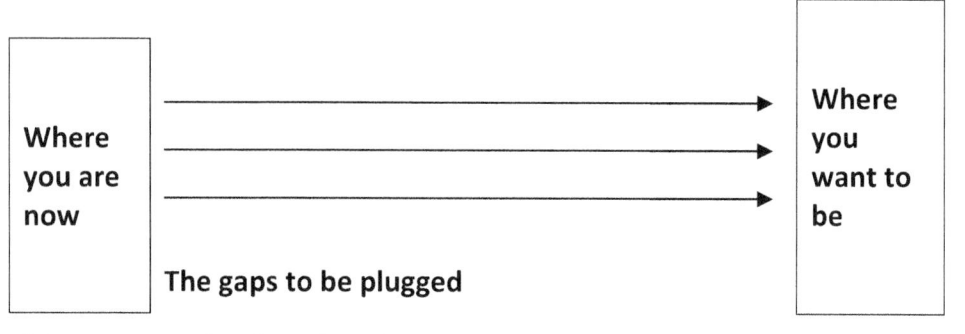

```
┌─────────┐                                    ┌─────────┐
│ Where   │  ─────────────────────────────▶   │ Where   │
│ you are │  ─────────────────────────────▶   │ you     │
│ now     │  ─────────────────────────────▶   │ want to │
│         │                                    │ be      │
└─────────┘                                    └─────────┘
             The gaps to be plugged
```

This exercise is hard work and requires a certain amount of insight from you. The detail in Box 7.1 might help guide you to complete such a gap analysis that you can view as underpinning your medical careers path and progression.

Box 7.1 Work out your own gap analysis

1. **Where you are now:** This will include a description of the important aspects of your work / home situation which are relevant to the goals that you envisage and changes you want to make. It may cover your strengths and weaknesses in your current role, your experience, your transferable skills, a review of how your current post measures up to your expectations and values. It might also include a SWOT analysis of your strengths, weaknesses, opportunities and threats (see Figure 7.4).

2. **Define your future career and other goals:** Be as specific as you can be about what you want to achieve. Describe your interests, areas of work and development you'd like to be responsible for or involved in, setting your wish to work in or type of role.
   Outline your aspirations and preferences. At this stage you can be as inventive or imaginative as you want to be. What would an ideal career progression look like?

3. **Describe the gap:** Compare items 1 and 2 and describe the main differences between your current state and your desired future position. Make a plan for change with timescales and milestones so that you can monitor progress. Discuss your plan with others who know you for a reality check. Outline the opportunities that might link where you are now with your future goals.

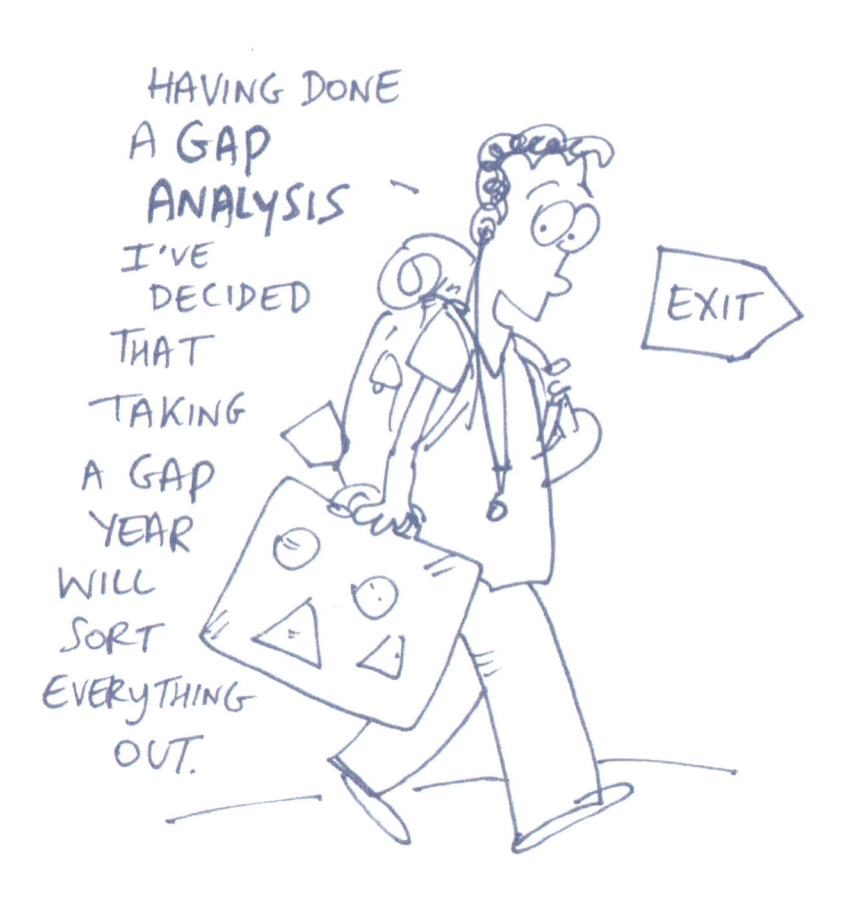

Try the Strengths, Weaknesses, Opportunities and Threats (SWOT) approach to review your current career path and medical role(s)

Strengths and weaknesses (or challenges) of your roles might relate to your clinical knowledge or skills, experience, expertise, decision making, communication skills, inter-professional relationships, political skills, timekeeping, organisational, teaching or research skills.

You should undertake a SWOT analysis of your own performance on your own, or with a group of colleagues. Brainstorm the strengths, weaknesses (or challenges), opportunities and threats of your situation using Figure 7.4 as a template.

Opportunities might relate to unexploited potential strengths, expected changes, options for career development pathways, hobbies and interests that could usefully be expanded.

Threats will include factors and circumstances that prevent you from achieving your aims for personal, professional and team development, and improvements in patient care.

A SWOT analysis creates opportunities to learn at the same time as undertaking the actual needs analysis.

Figure 7.4 SWOT analysis: how to do it

Strengths	Weaknesses
Opportunities	Threats

Complete each section - for example:
1. Strengths – what am I good at? What factors are in my favour?
2. Weaknesses – what am I not so good at?
3. Opportunities – what's likely to be useful that I could harness? What is happening that could help me? What is new, and is it good for me?
4. Threats – what could be a threat to my /our achievements? What's new and is it bad for me?

Prioritise important factors. Draw up goals and a timed action plan. Then consider:
- How can I optimise and extend the strengths identified?
- How can I minimise or overcome the weaknesses?
- How can I make most use of the opportunities?
- How can I avoid the threats or counter their effects?

And reflect on the next steps in the career path(s) you're considering – see Table 7.1 below:

Table 7.1 Reflection exercise: Career opportunity you are considering:

To what extent will this career opportunity:

	No............................Yes++
☐ Allow you to do the things you are good at and enjoy?	1　2　3　4
☐ Use your existing skills?	1　2　3　4
☐ Develop new skills which you wish to acquire?	1　2　3　4
☐ Give you what you want from work?	1　2　3　4
☐ Motivate you?	1　2　3　4

Be suitable for you in terms of:

☐ Location?	1　2　3　4
☐ Size of organisation?	1　2　3　4
☐ Work culture?	1　2　3　4
☐ Supervision (nature, extent, of you/by you)?	1　2　3　4

What else do you need to find out about this career opportunity?

Consider a portfolio career

A portfolio career describes how you might mix and match various posts. The *portfolio* description implies that the skills involved in the mix of jobs are transferable. It may be that you combine a number of clinical specialties or add in management, law, education, medical politics, academia, teaching, the media etc. Use the reflection exercise below in Box 7.2 to think more deeply about why you want to develop a portfolio career rather than stick single-mindedly with an unchanging career path.

Box 7.2 Reflection exercise: Consider how you would like to change features of your current job by converting to a portfolio career

This review exercise will help you to balance the mix of jobs you include in your future portfolio and what kind of mix of posts could make the change worthwhile. Consider:

- what it is that motivates you with your work – are there three key things?
- how satisfied you are with the amount of money you earn – do you want or need to earn more, can you manage on less income - taking your current outgoings into account?
- how content you are with the balance between your level of income and free time – how do you want to change the present balance?
- how often you use the range of your skills, knowledge and experience. Which of these do you want to develop or use more than in your present situation?
- do you want to develop a new interest or skill that will boost your creativity (research or a private business?), or job satisfaction (mentoring, teaching?)?
- how often you meet up with, or network with, like-minded colleagues – do you want to increase this part of your life, maybe take more interest in medical politics?

Anyone of any age and at any stage in their career may consider embarking on a portfolio career. You might be starting out in a regular post with other powerful interests that you want to develop – academic or competing in a sport, maybe. You might be a dissatisfied clinician in mid-career and be seeking variety and more expertise. You might be in your fifties and thinking of diversifying before retirement.

The strengths of a portfolio career are the flexibility, variety, personal development and ability to react to new opportunities or changing circumstances – either your personal ones or in relation to your practice or your NHS organisation. It is far better to seize the opportunities whilst you are on top of your job and starting to need variety and new challenges rather than wait until you are starting to burn out from a constant overload of work.

This may be your first opportunity to take stock of your career and try something different. You could include reasonably secure and well paid posts in your portfolio or take a risk. For example, as well as part-time general practice, you could retrain for another specialised area within or outside the health service or you could start a new business from scratch building on your health knowledge.

Be aware of your personal strengths, career and job preferences, motivation and priorities in life. Think how you want to balance time spent on work and leisure, and work and income. Understand what levels of responsibility, challenge and interaction with other people suit your personal style.

Try doing a SWOT analysis
You could undertake a SWOT analysis of your situation, working out the strengths, weaknesses, opportunities and threats (SWOT) as in Box 7.3. Doing the SWOT analysis with someone else can give you a more objective perspective.

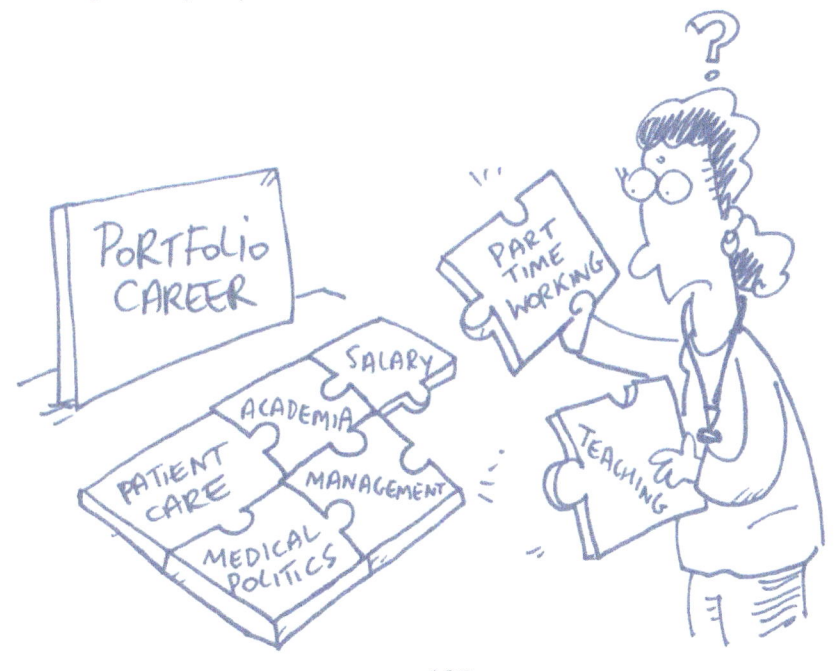

Box 7.3 SWOT analysis of you converting to a portfolio career

Possible strengths and opportunities of a portfolio career:
- potentially better paid part-time posts (e.g. expert posts)
- more time can be spent with colleagues (e.g. NHS politics, management, educational posts)
- flexible working enables you to fit in other commitments
- opportunities for creativity (e.g. educational post, writing, projects, leadership)
- combine work and hobby (e.g. travel, sports, writing)
- more public respect for your achievements (e.g. high profile post, project manager)
- instigate change (e.g. NHS politics, government post, project management)
- potentially increased job satisfaction and variety

Possible weaknesses and threats:
- reduced patient contact and less influence on decision making because of your lower profile in your current practice or organisation, may not suit you
- you may earn less in a non-clinical post
- as locum or sessional worker you may have no income whilst on holiday, or if you are sick or training
- financial insecurity
- seeking sessional or consultancy work continually can be personally draining
- making lesser contributions to NHS pension if in non-NHS post
- strain on your relationships with your partner or children maybe, if you travel away from home a lot or are focused on work even in your home life.

What attributes should you possess to make a success of a portfolio career?

Enthusiasm and interest are key. You need to be flexible and willing to take the risks involved, if you are giving up a secure full-time post. You will have to cope with change and uncertainty unless you settle quickly into regular work. Good time management is essential if you are going to juggle several diverse jobs.

It is easier to make a go of a portfolio career if you have an established expertise already that others seek. This might be a clinical expertise backed by a postgraduate qualification and experience or an educational qualification and background, for instance. You might be an experienced clinical facilitator who can transfer their skills between settings and challenges.

How to decide what options to explore

Reflect on what you are looking for from your work:
- the kind of work you enjoy – routine, exciting, prestigious
- the setting in which you want to work – community, hospital, rural, urban, travel
- the type of people for whom you want to care – ages and characteristics of patients
- the type of people with whom you want to work - whether in a small team or big organisation
- the extent of patient contact that suits you
- the level of income you consider (i) essential and (ii) desirable
- the working hours, holidays, study leave: how the hours fit with your current state and future domestic plans
- opportunities for parallel career interests such as research, writing, education, consultancy, private work or work related hobbies
- the extent of professional autonomy and responsibility you want
- in fact, your career anchors (see Chapter 5).

You should also take account of:
- the details of any training required – hours, practical difficulties, examinations
- the job prospects of alternative career paths: the opportunities for you to progress.

Then find out about the range of opportunities that match with what you want out of your portfolio career. Look out for job adverts in the usual way or local circulars. Seek out more careers information. Sound out people in your networks.

How much of the regular job should you give up – persuading your Trust or practice

Reducing to a part-time commitment may be difficult- others at work probably will not like any suggested change where you seem to be less available. Some full-time staff still scorn the part-time or assistant worker for 'shirking' the responsibility of full-time work. They might advertise for another part-time member of staff or arrange a job-share, appoint an advanced nurse practitioner with a different skill-mix in the team or make do with less doctor or manager time. Every Trust's or practice's circumstances will be different.

If you are a GP partner or other independent contractor with the NHS such as a medical consultant in private practice, you should establish a fair way of calculating the financial arrangements such that you keep externally earned pay for work done completely outside your core working hours in your own time, so long as the additional work does not impinge on the practice.

Good planning is key, so that you opt for a mix of jobs that suit you and end up with a portfolio of posts that together give you a fulfilling career. Anticipate any barriers that may impede your career progress or make the sustaining of your portfolio untenable. Work through the five point plan in Box 7.4 and adapt it as your own action plan.

Box 7.4 Five point action plan for making your portfolio career happen
1. Take stock – of the advantages and drawbacks
2. Review what opportunities there are
3. Match your abilities and circumstances to the job options
4. Negotiate with your manager or colleagues to reduce your current work commitment
5. Make a well considered change to your portfolio career

Making a career change – reflect, reflect, reflect

Questions to encourage your reflection on your career pathway and progression include:
- What do you think are the main strengths and weaknesses of your clinical practice?
- What do you think are your clinical care development needs for the future?
- What factors in your workplace or more widely, constrain you significantly in achieving what you aim for in your clinical work?
- What professional or personal factors significantly constrain you in maintaining and developing your skills and knowledge?
- (And more explicitly) How do you see your job and career developing over the next few years?

You may start to feel that your current job is getting in the way of being the kind of professional that you set out to be. The next two questions might enable you to see that there are specific, remediable factors that are getting in the way and you might choose to address them.

1. What do you think are the strengths and weaknesses of your relationships with patients?
An answer that suggests serious interpersonal difficulties, raises issues around developing a career away from a focus on clinical practice to laboratory based or research or teaching jobs, for instance. But if you have good interpersonal skills you may feel that a move to a job or role with more patient contact might be more rewarding.

2. What do you think are the main strengths and weaknesses of your relationships with colleagues?

Questions in this category can help if when you are contemplating a career change you realise upon reflection that it is more likely that it is the clash of personalities within your current workplace that is the base of your difficulties rather than the nature of the job itself.

Many established doctors develop portfolio careers that accommodate their desire to teach by negotiating a change in hours and search for a parallel teaching position, perhaps in a local university or for the Trust training and education department. Similarly they can become involved in research on a part-time basis, without it necessitating a major change in their career.

The model below in Figure 7.5 describes the stages in the cycle of change through which you might move as you progress along a career path and how you might be motivated to change.

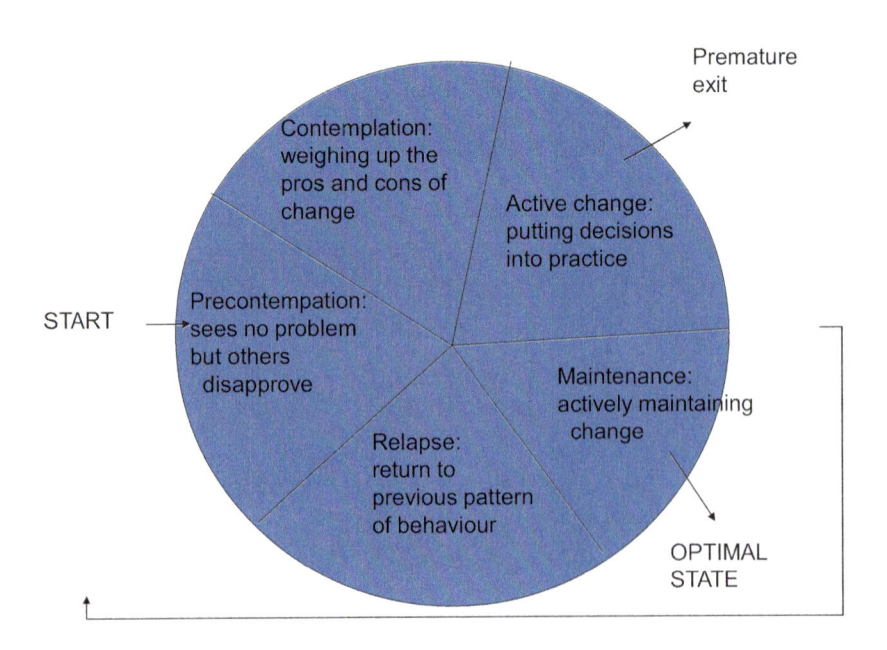

Figure 7.5 Cycle of career change

Individuals pass through the stage of contemplation and onto the stage of taking action for themselves. You should set realistic targets for that change that are achievable so as not to be demotivated if things don't go as well as you hoped ("I knew I couldn't do it!").

Change will not be possible unless those you are advising have thought through their career plan thoroughly, are committed to it and prepared to alter factors in your life so that it is possible to make the change happen in practice.

The GROW model

The GROW sequence is a simple way for you to consider change. This reflective exercise should help you to be specific about your career goals. The emphasis on realism will help you to be clear about your options and what is possible for you. Then you can decide what you are going to do and when. You might do this exercise on your own or with a coach or mentor.

Considering career change is never easy and this GROW approach starts with the positive; determining where you are trying to get to. Too often change starts with the problems and if you dwell on these barriers you may feel defeated before you have even started. If the change you are considering seems too big or too complex, you will need to begin with a small component of your goal, for example developing a particular skill or special interest.

Box 7.5 The GROW (Goal, Reality, Options, Way) approach for you to commit to a career plan of action

Step	Action (include timescales and milestones as appropriate)
Goal: Decide what you would you like to happen Decide what are your long term aims	

Reality: Assess what is really happening at the moment Review any problems: with your job, your organisation or practice, your specialism or your profession, your work/life balance Work out what is missing in your career or your life Beware of any assumptions you are making	
Options: Cover the full range of career or life choices you have and prioritise Brainstorm what different actions you could try to achieve your career goal	
Way forward: Plan which of these options you are going to do and how long it will take you and make a commitment	

Identify likely obstacles that might disrupt your plan and how to overcome them	
Seek support for your plan to increase the likelihood of it happening as you envisage	

Highlight your educational and development needs in your GROW plan in Box 7.5. Add timescales and milestones for your individual plan of action. Think how you will evaluate your progress and add those activities in too.

Overcoming Work Stress[3]

Stress is a pretty vague word that people interpret differently. Stress is the three way relationship between demands on a person, their feelings about those demands and ability to cope with the demands. A particular event or task can be stressful for you one day but not another - depending on how you're feeling and what other pressures are on you.

Work stress occurs when you've a heavy workload, your control over that work is limited, with too little support or help. You do need a moderate amount of stress though to perform well at work and maintain your zest for life. With zero stress you could be bored; but if you've too much stress over too long a period you'll likely get exhausted or burnt out.

Top stressors at work are insufficient time to complete tasks, frequent management reorganisations, lack of feedback about your effectiveness, bureaucracy++, and limited administrative support. Long unsociable hours at work can trigger stress and fatigue.

Stress affects your performance at work. As you become less able to carry out your work on time, your concentration gets worse, relationships may suffer if you're irritable and impatient, and you'll get further and further behind. You may suffer personal symptoms of stress too, such as anxiety, palpitations, insomnia, tire easily, lose your confidence, lack self-esteem and feel helpless.

It might be that if you can recognise that many of your difficulties and challenges at work are related to you feeling stressed and thus instigating your plans for a career change, you might settle into a stable career pathway if only you can overcome or minimise your work stress.

The kind of practical methods people can use to cope with stress at work are:
- seeking support from colleagues
- sharing problems with colleagues
- adopting better time management practices
- more appropriate booking times for appointments and meetings
- increased protected time off-duty, limiting working hours to those for which contracted
- admitting doubts and worries to others
- achieving a better balance between work and home commitments.

Avoiding the seven deadly sins of the workaholic is another good start to increased well-being and stress management:
1. Don't be a perfectionist.
2. Don't judge your mistakes too harshly.
3. Resist your desire to control everything.
4. Assertively decline requests to take on extra work or tasks if you are already pressed for time.
5. Look after your personal health and sustain your fitness.
6. Allow time for personal growth, your family and friends, and leisure activities.
7. Don't be too proud to ask for help – from colleagues, friends and family.

To stay on top of your career progression, you may need to regain your enthusiasm for learning and your quest for furthering your knowledge, skills and understanding. The personal satisfaction from completing a project, degree course or some other educational experience is likely to make any professional feel more fulfilled and to re-awaken their interest in all aspects of their work or seek further opportunities.

It is not stress itself that is the damaging factor but your inability to cope with it. In a changing world people need to learn new ways of coping and flourishing. That way lies survival.

In general stress management should include three approaches:
 (i)   **Thinking; for example:**
- Think more positively
- Put things in perspective and think longer-term
- Be more flexible
- Find ways to control your thinking style

 (ii)   **Behaviour; for example:**
- Talk about your worries to those at work who are responsible for the stress or are in a position to alleviate it
- Seek support from friends and family
- Be proactive about controlling stress provoking factors
- Be assertive
- Manage your time effectively

 (iii)   **Health; for example:**
- Achieve a better work-life balance
- Find methods of relaxation that work for you
- Follow a healthy lifestyle

So find out what help might be available to overcome your work stress – maybe an occupational therapist or counsellor – or sort out the management problems that have instigated the pressures on you with your line manager or team if you can. Then hopefully you will continue to progress along your chosen career path without any further changes being needed, if that suits you.

References
1. Chambers R, Mohanna K, Thornett A, Field S. *Guiding doctors in managing their careers.* Oxford: Radcliffe Publishing, 2006.
2. Chambers R (ed). *Career planning for everyone in the NHS - The Toolkit.* Oxford: Radcliffe Publishing, 2005.
3. Chambers R, Mohanna K, Chambers S. *Survival Skills for Doctors and their Families.* Oxford: Radcliffe Medical Press, 2003.

Chapter 8. Get ready, set, go............

Every doctor should be on a career pathway during the whole of their careers - not just at the beginning. There will be obstacles in your pursuit of a fulfilling career. Of course there will. But you can refuse to let those potential barriers control your decisions or actions. The main thing is to be aware which particular obstacle or challenge is yours. What are you up against here? What are you really afraid of? Are your fears rational? Are you maybe imagining a sequence like this - if you branch out into something new it will not work out, you will be unemployed and so you will not be able to pay the mortgage, so your partner will leave you? There are no guarantees in the pursuit of a particular job or role that really suits you except that once successful you will look back and wish that you had made the move a lot earlier.

Remember that there is likely to be a constant conflict in your inner-self between the part of you that wants and drives change and the part of you that resists it. There will be lots of things driving you to a goal such as your clinical interests and ambitions. There will also be things stopping you from pursuing that goal. But it's never too late to revise your career direction.

For you, trying to achieve a fulfilling career, there are many examples of major external factors beyond your control; such as the government shifting NHS priorities away from the special clinical interest area you have, or the illness of a colleague necessitating you taking on their basic work at the expense of working time spent on your special clinical interest area. Or maybe the hoped for support and co-operation you expected from others in your family or your colleagues at work is not there, if what you are proposing such as reducing your income or spending time away from your workplace gaining further skills or qualifications, will affect them too much. Their support (or not) will have a major effect on whether you are able to undertake many of the career development activities you plan.

As well as these unexpected factors that might spoil your plans, you may be assuming too much. It may be that you have insufficient knowledge and skills for the career development activities you envisage.

Or, you might not have fully anticipated the extent of qualifications, time or income or effort needed to implement your plans, for instance.

There may be other risks to your planned timetable too. You may not have thought through the consequences of your planned career evolution – such as how you will manage to do your everyday work as well as that of the new special clinical area, in line with your plans. Or you may not have predicted the new stress provoking factors that might arise from your revised weekly schedule when trying to fit in additional clinical work or studying for further qualifications.

But stay positive, keep going and find ways through if your career plans are reasonable and well thought out. Get what help & advice you can. You will face many decisions over the course of your working life, based on your changing needs along the way, many of which you would not have anticipated earlier on in your career when your personal and family life was different. Be prepared for frequent changes in your career plans and expectations as you move through Foundation and specialty training and build your career plans to overcome the challenges and make the most of the opportunities presented at each career transition – just as the medical students, junior and senior doctors did who shared their career histories in Chapter 1.

And finally

Here's a checklist of seven steps[1] to really crystallise the actions you can take.

Step 1 – Know yourself
- Review and update your CV. It is a snapshot of your career.
- Reflect on what makes you tick, your leadership and decision making styles, extent to which you are a team player.
- Be clear about what is important to you in your career.

Step 2 – Know what you want
- How much of a challenge you want.
- How much you want to follow other people's guidance or lead.
- How much money you want or need.
- What kind of work/life balance suits you.

Step 3 – Know where you are
- Have a good understanding of your achievements and skills.
- Know your strengths and weaknesses.
- Understand what your career anchors are.

Step 4 – Know where you want to go
- Check out the options and opportunities open to you.
- Compare what is on offer with your responses to steps 1 & 2 above.

Step 5 – Know the gap
- Analyse the gap between where you are now and the variety of options for where you want to be.

Step 6 – Know how to get there
- Have a range of strategies to bridge that gap in your career plan.
- Develop a realistic action plan with contingencies for if or when your ideal career path does not work out.

Step 7 – Get support
- Find a mentor.
- Develop a network outside your immediate colleagues of others who are or could be important to you or informative about your future career.

Make your realistic plan

Assess how ready you are to change career, take forward your current career plan, create a new business - plot the resources you'll need – complete the *What, Where, When, How?* column in Table 8.1. Identify the gaps so you can begin to build an action plan to identify your resource needs to be successful and achieve your goals.

Table 8.1 Compile your in-depth forward looking medical career plan[2]		
Symbol	Infrastructure/resources you'll need?	What, Where, When, How?
	Qualifications (University – postgraduate e.g. master's, CPD, local or national qualifications)	
	Location of medical posts (nearby or travel or relocate?)	
	Money/earnings (pay scale, NHS or private work etc. full or part-time?)	
	Expertise (skills, knowledge, capability, competence)	
	People conversations (careers mentor, supervisor, colleague)	
	Specialty/foci (develop specific expertise/interest)	
	Information technology (digital transformation of care and delivery; online networks)	
	Communication (e.g. professional networks; social media)	
	Time for self (regular exercise, hobbies, 'down' time, family time)	
	Other: special interests e.g. professional, allied	
	Other: achievements you hope for e.g. reducing inequalities; expert skills	

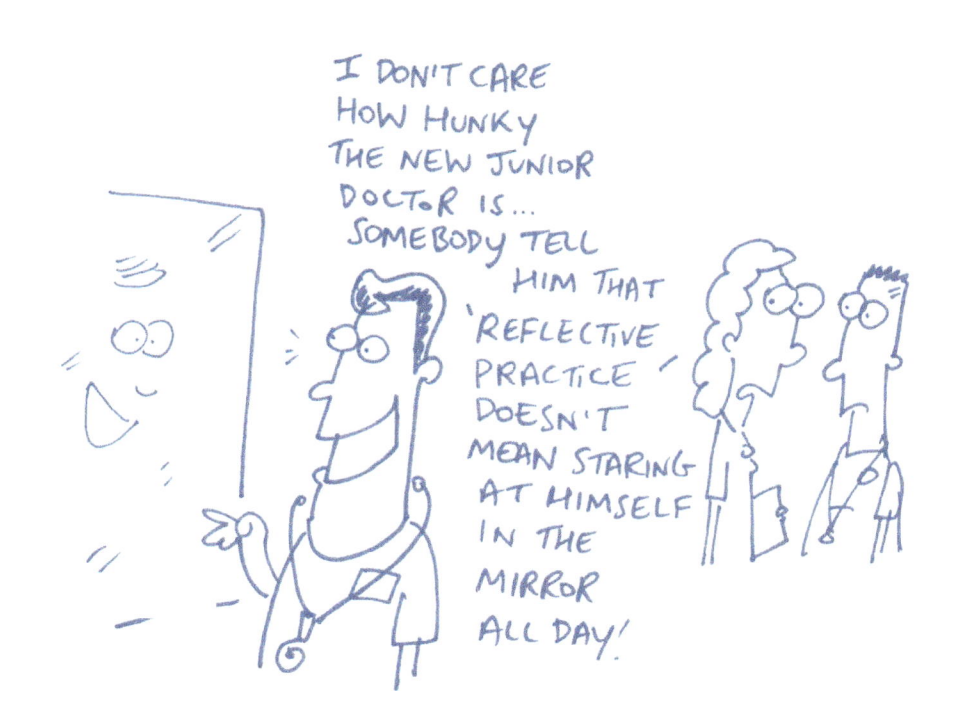

Your career compass[1,2]

So having read much of the material in this book that's relevant to you, have a go at completing your career plan – for now; in One year's time; then in Five year's time.

A. Who are you and where are you now?

A.1 Looking inwards

Consider:
(i)   You
- What are your strengths and weaknesses in your various roles or posts?
- Do you understand your own personality: have you undertaken a personality profile test? Do the insights about your personality affect your career choice?
- What transferable skills do you have that might fit you for a different kind of career?
- How does your current work and life measure up to your inner values?

- What kind of roles and responsibilities do you prefer? Do you enjoy leading or following? Do you like to manage or be managed?
- What fears do you have that you need to overcome?
- What qualities do you have that you need to exploit or harness?

(ii)   Your current job
- Do the features of your job fit with your personal style?
- How satisfied are you with your job – working hours, responsibility, location, patient contact, workload, income, challenge, opportunities for change or development, extent of socialising, your skills, on-call commitment, support from colleagues, variety?
- How satisfied are you with your career in general?
- What aspects of work do you value?
- Are there inner barriers that hinder your career advancement in your current job (e.g. self-doubt, low self-esteem)?
- Do you act the part in your post, even if you do not feel confident?
- Do you exceed your job description? You can impress others with your initiative and capability.
- Do you set yourself new targets within your job to keep your interest alive and provide new challenges?
- Do you nurture your relationships with other colleagues? You never know when you may need their support or help.

A.2 Looking outwards
Consider:
- What opportunities are there for promotion or other roles or extending your skills, in your current job?
- What opportunities might there be for developing new skills or enhancing current skills in your present job?
- What other jobs are on offer elsewhere for which you might apply?
- What other role(s) and responsibilities do you see yourself taking on?
- Have you got enough support from others at work?
- What qualities and skills do others perceive that you have?
- Is your potential recognised or realised in your current post?

A.3 Looking sideways

Consider:
- How do your current workload and conditions impact on your family and other aspects of your non-working life?
- How satisfied are you with your lifestyle and time spent outside work – sport, relaxation, hobbies, travel?
- How much quality time do you have for friends and family?
- What is the balance like between your current work and other aspects of your life?
- Do you have a mentor or adviser? A role model or influential colleague might well give your career a boost.

Box 8.1 What makes you think about possibly leaving your current post?
- What do you dislike about your current job?
- Is it boredom, stress, work overload, relationships, the environment?
- How are these problems affecting you, specifically?
- What would you like to do less of in your job?
- What would you like to do more of?
- Have you been here before? Is the problem part of a pattern in your career?
- What will you be looking for in your next job or way of life if you leave?

B. What changes do you want to make?

Consider:
- To what extent are you content to remain in the same job, specialty, practice or NHS Trust?
- To what extent will your current role satisfy you in one / three years time?
- What is it that you most want to achieve? What are your career goals?
- Do your career goals conflict with other types of success or fulfilment that you are seeking in other areas of your life (for instance, financial goals, social goals, leisure goals, personal goals in relation to your family)?

- What will be your strengths and skills and achievements by certain time milestones?
- How will you acquire those skills and experience in the meantime to develop your full potential? Skills developed outside work may be just as important as those developed as part of your job.
- What resources do you have to help you achieve your career goals?
- Consider applying for promotion to show others that you are motivated to progress your career.

B.1 Where do you want to be in ONE year's time?

Write down your goals after reading through the career challenges in Box 8.2

Box 8.2 Take a career challenge in formulating your goals
What role do you see yourself doing in three, five, fifteen years time? Think widely: academic career, research interest or audit, opportunities for teaching, location, preferences or hobbies, access to relatives, alternative and parallel clinical or management work, availability of cover by colleagues, supportive colleagues, sponsors and friends. Do you know of someone whose career pathway or roles you would like to emulate?

Looking inwards

-
-
-

Looking outwards

-
-
-

Looking sideways

-
-
-

B.2 Where do you want to be in FIVE year's time?

Write down your goals:

Looking inwards

-
-
-

Looking outwards

-
-
-

Looking sideways

-
-
-

C. How are you going to get there?

Work out the series of steps you will need to take over the next twelve months to achieve your one year goals; and longer-term action for your five year or even ten or fifteen year goals. Think how to make things happen. To whom can you talk to get more information or advice? Who can you visit to see if their type of work appeals to you? Who can give you well informed careers guidance or career counselling? How can you gain the preliminary achievements and experience that you need?

C 1 *Getting ready to make a change*: What do you need to do first?

- Further reflection and review of how satisfied you are with your career, your job, your life in general – as in Stages A.1 and A.2 and A.3.
- Discuss your satisfaction and options with others close to you – at home, your family and friends, work colleagues, trusted advisers and confidantes.
- Find out more information and facts about other careers or new skills.
- Ask someone for advice about opportunities in their field or specialty and what their jobs entail.
- Seek further careers information, careers advice or guidance.
- Make a list of your options and reflect (with someone whose opinion you value) on their relative advantages.

C 2 *Are you ready to change?*
- How positive are you about going ahead and making changes?
- Does what you are proposing fit with your ethics, values and boundaries?
- What is it that has limited you from making changes in the past? Have you overcome those constraints or barriers now?
- Are you clear about what interests and motivates you to work effectively?

C 3 *So what will you do?* Make your plans happen with timetabled action. Think of:
- Setting goals
- What new insights, knowledge, skills and attitudes you need to develop
- Using your skills and experience
- Your timetable
- How you will proceed
- Support and resources you will need to make your plans come to fruition
- Overcoming limiting factors – what risks you need to manage
- Situations you may wish to influence – to prevent or provoke events or activities.

D. What will you do if you don't get what you want or hope for?

Write down your contingency plans: for instance:
- How could you change your current job so that you have more job satisfaction?
- Re-evaluate your options. What is your 'second choice' alternative career path or career development?
- Re-assess your previous goals and objectives.
- What other skills might you develop within medicine or in your leisure time?
- Could you get more balance into your life by building in more self-development time?
- Think again if anyone else might help you through all your networks and contacts.
- Can you fit two different jobs into your life, working part-time on each?
- Think again about what you really want out of life.
- Counter any self-defeating beliefs that you have uncovered in undertaking the review of your career.
- Adopt some better personal stress management in all sections of your life and work.
- Build up your support mechanisms – at work, with friends, with family and your partner at home.

That's it then – get ready, set, go..

References
1. Chambers R (ed). *Career planning for everyone in the NHS - The Toolkit.* Oxford: Radcliffe Publishing, 2005.
2. Garcarz W, Chambers R, Ellis S. *Make your healthcare organisation a learning organisation.* Oxford: Radcliffe Medical Press, 2003.

Printed in Great Britain
by Amazon